WAIT, Don't Take My Uterus

Geoffrey Charles Cly, MD, FACOG

DEDICATION

I dedicate this book to:

Mom & Dad, I miss you. I love you. Thank you for being around me during the times I've needed you the most. I hope to see you again someday.

Megan, my wife, my Beautiful, you have been my strength and support from the beginning of this endeavor. I am so thankful we are in this journey together. I couldn't have done this without you. I love you!

To all my kids, Geoffrey, Brooklyn, Marcus, Mia, Christian, and Victoria, I love you all. I hope and pray you will seek happiness and find joy in your lives. You guys are the joy and happiness in my life.

To ALL my Patients, I am so honored to have been trusted as your doctor. You are like family to me. I often wonder how or why destiny decided our hearts and souls should intertwine over the years, but in the end, it has been your prayers, love, and support that gave tremendous meaning to my life. I am grateful for you and may God Bless you always.

CONTENTS

ACKNOWLEDGMENTS

Megan, you are my wife, my love, my young hottie, my strength and I thank you for patience while an old man like me finds quiet space away from the kids to get this book finished. You always give more and love more than asked for. I love you!

Geoffrey Jr., Brooklyn, Marcus, Mia, Christian, and Victoria, my children. I am so thankful that I am able to remember all your names because there are so many of you. I expect you will take the autographed copy of this book that I am going to give to you and you will place it in a box or closet and not read it for many, many years until after I am gone. So when that day comes, and you come across this message, know that I love you and I expected you to chuckle and say, "Daaaaad you're not funny" and know that I am laughing right now as I write this.

Tony Cly, and Jeannie Breitenbach, my brother and sister. I love you and I have enjoyed the closeness that we have and I couldn't have gotten through everything with Mom and Dad without you guys. Love you.

Rusty 'Pops' Richardson, my father-in-law, thank you for all your patience and wisdom over the past couple years and for helping out soooo many times at the house while I was writing and working on the website. Megan and I couldn't have done this without your support.

Kathy Powell, my same age aunt in-law, you have been behind the scenes helping us with those wild animals we call children! Oh my gosh without you helping Megan and I when we went on conferences and worked on things we would have probably lost our minds!

Denise Zeitler, Aunt Barb Richards, Walter Radloff, Angie Cly, Ryan Breitenbach, and Nicole Cato (placed in order of wisdom years accumulated) thank you for helping with the kids while Megan and Kathy were away when I was writing the book. Thank you for bringing your kids over to distract my kids when I was writing. Thank you for taking the wild animals on weekends or to the "Man Store" so Megan and I could get away. And lastly, I thank one of you for indirectly, accidentally being responsible for Obamacare and all the subsequent healthcare complexities as well as keeping America safe.

Barb Lomont it was you who gave my kids healthy food while my wife was away when all I had given them was fast food. Thank goodness you and Maddie had enough energy to babysit and distract Christian and Vicky while I left and wrote part of this book in the Leo Park parking lot.

'Brother' Tom Biesiada, my spiritual advisor and early editor of the Pocket Guides. Without your guidance and prayerfulness I might have started another protestant reformation church called The Clytherean Church, lol. Thank you for bringing me back down to earth so I could focus on getting this book out to the world.

Megan Uphoff you have incredible insight. You called it early on, "It is going to show up differently than you can imagine", and how right you were! Thank you for being my friend, my office nurse, preop & postop surgery nurse, a kind ear in L&D, and helping me and assisting me on the background details as we put all this together. I hope to have you part of this journey as it grows through the years.

Paul and Rebecca Harrington, we go way, way back. Rebecca, thank you for bringing Paul in to the office, even though he talks for you AND everyone else. He is the Jedi, I am the Padawan, and you are his Princess Leia. Your trust and assistance through the years has been invaluable.

Joni Blomeke you are an amazing woman and mother. Your smile and joyful outlook on life is contagious. Through the years I always knew it was going to be a good day when I saw your name.

Michael Silvers, from Warrior Camp forward, your encouragement and solid pushes have helped me go to the edge of my comfort zone and achieve big things. I feel like we are just warming up, the Big Stuff is yet to come!

Brad Lomont and Casey O'Boyle I am still not sure why I called you two bozos back in 2003 when we formed Rekindle The Fire. It must have been The Holy Spirit that made me do it. You guys didn't directly help with the book, but you old farts get a mention on this page because you would routinely screen my calls and send me to voice mail at which time I would rant and rave and curse your names but it allowed me to de-stress and get my frustrations out at your expense, so for that I thank you both greatly.

Amélie Hoeferle, oh my goodness! It is like you were sent from above. I had given up on being able to get this book finished by the deadline. I had accepted my fate, and all of a sudden you appeared and saved the day. Thank you so much for your editing and assistance in putting these pieces together so we could meet the deadline and get this book completed and published!

Jolene Reault your help with the graphics, media posts, and book cover was amazing. You've got a ton of talent and I am so thankful for your patience, kindness, and expertise.

So many thanks for you Angel Tuccy. You have been such an amazing help in this entire journey. I am writing this book because it was you who finally made me see the light about becoming an author. I am so grateful to you for your guidance with the press releases, the marketing, the book training, and your patience with my temper tantrums. Actually what touched me the most is when you were worried about me during my darkest days recently and made me promise to talk to you in a few days because of how low I really was. (I was worried about me as well) Without you I don't know what could have happened, thank you from the bottom of my heart for believing in me and encouraging me to write this book.

Brigitta Hoeferle, I don't know where to begin. Well, let me honestly say this, my wife frequently says, "Well, what does Brigitta think?" That says something about your wisdom right there. I am so thankful for you. Your guidance and wisdom have propelled me to new levels of existence that would not have been possible. Everytime I have a catastrophe or major problem in my life you always see the answer and the path for me to conquer it. Your graceful wisdom flows out of you like a beacon from a lighthouse shining the way home.

Adam Markel you gave me the insight to realize that if I wanted a different result I had to do something different that was at the edge of my comfort zone. After that realization, you showed me how to find the courage and become unstoppable. And lastly, your example and book, "Pivot", showed me the way. My life is forever changed because of your mentorship, I will always be grateful to you.

Gerry Foster when I first met you in Martha's Vineyard on the shore where we kayaked I knew you were the real deal. Your joyfulness and happiness got you "in trouble" with Adam Markel. The way you responded to him "chiding" you was an example of humble wisdom and courageous leadership. You impressed me that day and also in the way you helped me create the branding for HonestOBGyn.com. I could not have tapped into the emotions and "blue ocean" without you.

Bill Walsh, when you said your information was going to come out like a firehose you weren't kidding. In 2 days at your Rainmaker program I received the equivalent of a college semester of business information. After that, I was hooked and I knew I had to be part of Powerteam International. I also told my wife afterwards that, Bill Walsh IS the superconductor engine that rockets a business into space. I thank you and look forward to what is coming next with you.

Ken and Bill Courtright, your company The Income Store, Sean Kavanaugh, and the people who have worked on the website along this journey have made this process memorable. I have learned so much along the way. For that I thank you.

There have been so many more people who have been a part of this journey. I am thankful for all of you. I know I probably missed some of you. If I didn't mention you, please know that I value you and what you have done for me. Also, if you buy a hard copy of the book I will gladly personally sign it for you ;-) (that is a little wink, wink symbol)

Foreword:

When I met Dr. Geoff Cly in 2012 we were fellow
students, taking part in a self-development group. We
later joined the same Global Mastermind Program
which gave us many opportunities to work together
closely. He always stood out – in a very good way:
Not stuck up or self-absorbed, like many other white-
coated doctors I know. Always humble, ready to learn
more. Vulnerable and strong – all at the same time.
Geoff is funny! He doesn't take himself too seriously
and yet, he takes his job – no, his calling – very
seriously: Giving women and those close to them
options. Options and choices around healing, options
around how to solve recurring health issues specific
to women, and options for education. Specifically for
education on the most common and recurring female
medical conditions.
He could easily diagnose a woman with the most
expensive treatment and make a bundle of money by
misusing the power of his degree and expertise. He
doesn't, though. And this is what sets him apart from
many others in his field. Dr. Cly is not that kind of man
and not that kind of doctor. He is, in fact, the honest
OB/Gyn who is more passionate about giving his
patients the best options, not his bank account. A
philosophy that speaks louder than words.
Dr. Cly cares. He is a kind and funny dad to his
children. He is a caring and providing husband to his
wife, Megan. And he was a caring son to his late
mother and father who, essentially, continue to be the
"why" behind his actions. Of all the doctors I've dealt
with throughout my lifetime, Dr. Cly is the only one
who truly meant what he said when he declared his
hippocratic oath.

Geoff chose me as his professional and personal coach in late 2014. Although my clients are mainly women in C-level positions, he is one of my male legacy clients and I am exceptionally proud, excited, and humbled to be a part of his success story. He gave me the privilege of leading and guiding him, mentally, emotionally, educationally, and sometimes even spiritually.

I speak with his permission when I say that Geoff has often times questioned his journey as he was taking leaps of faith into the unknown. Nevertheless, he was always vulnerable enough to ask for guidance and he was driven enough to push through and step outside his comfort zone. And, wow, did he ever step out of his comfort zone!

Dr. Cly started building an educational website "HonestOBGyn.com," designed particularly to address the everyday questions, problems, and symptoms the thousands of patients in his practice bring to him. How many doctors do you know who do that? He takes the time to listen to each of his patients individually, to address their concerns, and to give personalized advice.

The journey of building this website and the different challenges which came with that helped shape him into the person he is today. Geoff did not buy into any doubt or negative self-talk, nor did he accept his own emerging small-mindedness when he questioned his self-worth.

Instead, Dr. Cly chose to risk losing his position at his local hospital for his clients, no, for ALL women around the world. His vision for humanity was bigger than holding on to a steady paycheck! He knew it took somebody to take action for the medical injustices he encountered day after day. Geoff accepted the calling to educate women about their rights, their choices, and their responsibilities for their bodies. Often, solutions to female medical issues do not require a surgical knife, expensive prescription drugs, or endless visits to the doctor's office. They require women to have the necessary information to make educated decisions for themselves and their bodies. The biggest "why" behind what Dr. Cly is doing is a family trauma you'll read about in one of the first chapters. It is the reason why he keeps re-investing the money he makes as a physician into providing expert advice to all women – not only his patients. It wasn't easy for Geoff to revisit this part of his past. Yet, he pushed through it – for you! He isn't stuck in a victim role, he is a victor. And he wants women around the world to be victresses, too. He wants you to be empowered champions of your self-determined health.

Dr. Geoff Cly, the Honest OB/Gyn, has many fans. You may already be one of them. And if not, prepare to be one very soon! Enjoy this book, gift it to as many women, husbands, fathers, daughters, mothers, grandmothers as you possibly can!
Geoff has now given birth himself: to this book – for you. What a great experience it is to bring life, with all the waves of excitement, anxiety, euphoria, and stress. What a great legacy it is to bring options and solutions to a society, that thinks they're only part of a system.
Dr. Cly honestly cares.
Enjoy and pass along.

Of service,

Brigitta Hoeferle
CEO NLP Institute of Atlanta

WAIT! Don't Take My Uterus!

Introduction to: *WAIT, Don't Take My Uterus*

Wait, Don't Take My Uterus is a book for women that unveils the truth on OBGyn secrets, how to avoid unnecessary surgery, and how to make sure that they are on the best path to feeling and healing their best. This book blends 20 years of experience as a board-certified OBGyn along with medical knowledge, in order to help guide women. Along the way, stories will be told from 20 years of medical experience; Some of them funny, some of them shocking, some of them sad. My goal is to empower women and guide them while providing transparency into the medical field from the eyes of an OBGyn.

This book isn't only about the truth of the Women's health industry and revealing the ugly medical secrets that are not being told to patients. It is also about me, Dr. Geoffrey Cly, and my own story – how my journey has been progressing over the last 20 years. How my tragedies, losses, successes, and discoveries have altered the way I look at medicine and improved how I treat patients. Ultimately, it is about how I can make a difference in people's lives and how that can change yours.

The idea for this book was initially planted many years ago and then just recently in the last couple of years solidified into a reality. I realized that I had to tell all women in the world about the truth, in order to make a difference and to help them. And I realized that continuing to only teach doctors and attempt to guide doctors on doing what is "right" was not working. The doctors in almost every community who are hiding behind their medical degrees and not telling patients the full truth about unnecessary surgeries – among other problems – caused my frustration to skyrocket. I could no longer turn a blind eye to doctors who were choosing surgeries or treatments based on financial gain and not what is truly best for their patients. I finally understood the only way patients can avoid being forced into unnecessary surgeries or inappropriate treatments is that they have to know the details about their treatment choices. They should be able to have a list of ALL available treatments not just the individual one their particular doctor decided upon for them. When the patients are informed and then realize a doctor is not doing what is best for them, they will go elsewhere. When patients know what to ask for and know about different treatments, they will go to doctors who are doing what is in their best interest. Transparency and knowledge by patients about current treatments is what will improve the medical system. Additionally, when a doctor realizes he/she is losing patients because he/she is out of date or not offering appropriate treatments, that doctor has a choice to make; do what is right for the patient, or eventually go out of business.

1 My Dad, a Happy Lazy Drunk

The first time I realized as a doctor that I could not trust other physicians was after my first experience with a family member: my dad. The tragedy and the suffering that we went through after this experience is what really started to change my thought process.

My dad was 56 years old and he was a man who had struggled with alcohol his whole life. In his last several years, he had tried to kick alcoholism and attempted to straighten out, but was not able to. I would describe my dad as the happy, lazy drunk. What I mean by that is that he didn't get violent, he didn't lay a finger on any of us. He wasn't verbally abusive, but he was the kind of alcoholic who would drink at the end of the day and maybe during work and then come home and pass out in his easy chair. He wouldn't really yell at us kids too much, but he wasn't there as a father either. As a result of the alcoholism, my parents got divorced when I was 12. I was the oldest of three, with a younger brother and sister. As you can imagine, due to the alcohol in my father's life, we didn't have many fantastic father-son moments. The times I can remember going out with my dad, he was drinking; there was always a cup in the car that was filled with alcohol, and he always ended up falling asleep at random moments. The alcoholism was his challenge in life, and that challenge continued through his life until the age of 59.

He was working as a carpet salesman and the alcoholism was affecting that too, since he was drinking on the job. His boss called me and said, "Hey, I'm gonna fire your dad if he doesn't stop drinking." Subsequently, the boss and I ended up holding an intervention for him.

At this point in 1998 I was an OBGyn Resident Physician. I graduated medical school in 1996. I was in my second year of a four year OBGyn residency training program at Wright State University School of Medicine OBGyn Residency Training program. I was busy, but also, as a doctor an intervention was something I had heard about and I wanted to help my own dad as well. And so I helped: I helped organize an intervention for my dad. I wanted to give him a chance to heal himself. The intervention was successful in the sense that he agreed to go inpatient for alcohol treatment. He was even able to go into the Veterans Hospital inpatient program since he served in the Navy years earlier. Unfortunately, the whole detox attempt ultimately did not work out. He did end up doing a couple of treatments and some outpatient therapy, but just was not able to kick alcohol or stop drinking. However he did manage to get other jobs.

While I was in Residency, for the next 2 years, we lived about an hour and a half apart from each other. At this point, here I was, a young doctor, trying to have a relationship with my father who was an alcoholic for longer than I had been alive. I realized I had "passed" him mentally, emotionally, and developmentally as well, all because of the alcoholism. So, we were as close as we could be given that he was drinking every night. I loved my dad, and I soon realized that his capacity for a relationship with me was limited by his alcohol consumption. I accepted it though, and loved him through it at the level that he was able to love me back. For the next year or so I helped my dad through different processes and events. I was able to take time to go visit him and tried to help him as much as possible. Eventually, he landed a job as a Sears Department store salesman.

I remember it was 1999, I was a chief resident (which was my last year of OBGyn residency) when I got a call from dad and he said, "Hey son, I think I, I need to go to the doctor. I'm coughing and I think I have an infection." He described the symptoms to me and based on what he was describing to me, I said, "Dad, it sounds like you have congestive heart failure and it sounds more like your heart isn't pumping effectively, You're getting fluid back up in your lungs." I didn't think it was an infection and I suggested he go to the VA Hospital near Lancaster, Ohio and tell the ER doctors that I sent him there. I wanted them to look for CHF, or congestive heart failure, and he ended up agreeing to go. A day or so later that week he went to the doctor and called me after his appointment and said, "I went to the doctor and told them what you said – they all laughed and asked what does the obstetrician gynecologist know about heart failure? They told me that it's just bronchitis and then gave me some Erythromycin and said I'll be fine." My dad went on to tell me that they did a chest X Ray and evaluated him. He was chuckling and laughing at the comments they made and said that they were teasing him and stating that I should just stick to my own field and not try to assess other areas of the body. Of course, I was relieved that it was only something minor but I couldn't shake the feeling that it actually sounded like congestive heart failure. We hung up the phone from that conversation and I thought to myself, "Man, maybe, I don't know what I'm talking about. Maybe I am not a very good physician."

Unfortunately, several days later, one of the worst things happened. Even though I have talked about it over and over for the past 20 years, it still chokes me up to this day. I was in the middle of performing a Cesarean section when I got a message from one of the nurses. They told me my wife was on the phone and that she wanted to talk to me about my dad. I replied abruptly with something along the lines of "Oh, it's probably about his drinking again. Just tell her that I will call her back after the C-section is over." Thinking back, I believe we had just delivered the baby and we were closing the uterus; so it wasn't the optimal time to break away. However, my attending physician was in the room and told me I needed to take the call and then he scrubbed in and had everything under control. Naturally, I thought that was unusual, but when my attending tells me to go do something, I do it. I went outside to take the phone call and the nurse said, "Okay, Dr. Cly, it'll be on line one." So I went into a private room to take the phone call, that's when the worst news that I could imagine came over the phone to me. I said, "Hey, what's going on? What's going on with dad?" I just remember my wife saying something to the effect of, "It's not good, they found him this morning in his apartment and he passed away in his sleep."

"What! Oh God no!, Nooo, nooo, nooo," It felt as if something had sucked the air from my lungs and punched me very hard in my chest at the exact same time. This news completely devastated and shocked me. It was something that no one ever wants to hear, let alone without any warning. I sat in that small room and dropped to the floor and just cried, cried uncontrollably for what felt like an eternity. I know part of the reason was because deep down inside my heart and soul at that moment, I knew he died of a heart attack due to congestive heart failure and I knew that I had failed my dad. I knew I was right in my diagnosis even though the doctors said otherwise. And I felt like a huge failure as well as so guilty because I let my dad die and what kind of a son and doctor would allow that to happen.

From that point on, my ability to trust doctors was deeply affected. At the same time, I felt completely responsible for my dad's death, and I felt that I failed him as a son. And even 20 years later, I still think that if only I had been there or only had driven to take him to the doctor, taking the day off of work, that he might still be alive. People have told me over the years that it wasn't my fault, but still deep down inside I know I could have made a difference, I had the right diagnosis. I knew what was going on, but I doubted myself and I doubted myself because of other doctors who didn't care as much as I did and didn't know my dad as much as I did. As a result of that, I lost my dad that day. That was the moment that changed the way I treated my own patients and the way I look at all patients.

Over the years I've found time and time again that there are doctors who do not care much and do not take the time with their patients that they need to. I have built my practice by taking care of people, making sure that I treat them like I would treat my family, making sure that I protect them and help them heal from the condition that they are having, and to ultimately protect them from other doctors who don't care as much. If I have to, I'll stand up to doctors, I'll make a comment or go against other doctors if it's in the best interest of the patient. It's gotten me in trouble a little bit but all of my colleagues and medical directors have always said that the things I do are out of the best interest for the patients, even when I'm ruffling feathers. And that's really because of the tragedy that I went through. That my family went through. That began when my dad passed away.

2 Not My Mom! - "Why God, Why Would You do this???"

The next thing that happened really changed my world and changed the way I think about life and people. This event forever changed the way I live my life and the core of who I have become. In order for you to understand who I am and how this affected me, I want you to understand where I came from and a little bit about my early years. As a result of my parents divorce when I was twelve and being the oldest kid in the family, I was kind of "the man of the house" growing up. I received a lot of responsibility early on, more responsibility than some kids get. This helped shape me and form what would become the person I am today. As I went through my teenage years and early, early adulthood, I was a mama's boy. Yes, and I am proud of it. I love my Mom. She was the breadwinner since my dad was an alcoholic and really wasn't able to support or provide any financial care for us.

During my teenage years after the divorce, I was distant from him for a couple of years because of everything going on and it was then that I got really close to my Mom. Now, that doesn't necessarily mean that I was always the easiest kid. Although she was my main support and parent, I still was a stubborn, independent thinking, and sassy teenager. Even so, she was the person I would go to, the person who gave me love and support, the person who would keep encouraging me to move forward. She was so proud of me. In college, as an 18 year old freshman at the University of Dayton, when I switched from Pre-Law to Pre-Med she was surprised but very supportive.

That story is in my HonestOBGyn Facebook videos. A lot of people are very surprised about the reason I became an OB/Gyn instead of a lawyer. The day that I changed my major from Pre-Law to Pre-Med was the day I saw something so incredible and jaw dropping that I instantly knew my destiny was to become an OB/Gyn.

Later, when I was in medical school, she would tell everybody that her son was going to be a doctor and she was one of the proudest mothers I could imagine having. One of the things she used to do was to call me and say, "Hey, Geoff, I got a question for you. I have some pain... or I have these symptoms... What do you think they are?" Even when I was in med school, like in the first week, she's asking me things I had no idea about because I just started. But she would always do that, it was kind of her fun thing I knew I could expect from her. Over the years of med school and residency, she would then start talking to other people about me and that led to her offering to ask me medical questions on their behalf. Then she would call me and explain their symptoms and go back and offer my answers and expertise to them as if she was one of my medical nurses.

Mom was a very outgoing person. She was able to strike up a conversation with anyone. She would give anyone the shirt off her back and she just had a way about her that made people feel comfortable. She was always able to see the person in the corner of the room, who was not part of the group. Everytime, she would automatically just reach out to them and make sure they were included in whatever was going on. She had a big heart.

As I mentioned above about her offering to ask me questions for people she knew, I later realized this was just another example of her selfless behavior and a way she could try to help others who were suffering and offer her kindness to them. I used to get frustrated that she would ask her friends and coworkers or they would ask her and she would say, sure, I'll ask Geoff. Then she'd call me and say, "Hey, Geoff Hey, what'd you think about this? So-And-So is having this and this and these problems. What do you think it is? What should they do?" I usually responded with: "I have no idea, Mom. I have to keep studying or working Mom. I got to go, I can't, you know, I can't do this, I don't have time." So for a long time she would do that. She knew it drove me crazy, but at the same time she was so proud of me for becoming a doctor.

I was in private practice for about a year/year and a half. She called me one day during private practice office hours when I was seeing patients. I was busy seeing patients, busy trying to grow the practice, and during the daytime with patients waiting, I don't have a lot of time for phone calls, but she called me and said, "Hey Geoff, I'm having these weird symptoms. What do you think they are?" and I was like, "Mom, I don't know what they are. I'm not sure." I finally asked "what's going on?" She said, "I'm having these buzzing sensations and, and kind of electrical sensations in my head, kind of flashing lights." I asked her some questions and said "Mom, I have no idea what that is. I really don't, could you talk to your doctor and see what he thinks?" She said, okay, I'll do that. She went to her family doctor and told him the symptoms and told him that I had told her to go there and she called me back a short time later and said, "Geoff, I talked to him. He thinks everything's okay. He thinks it's probably hypoglycemia. He gave me some things to try and some glucose tablets to make sure my blood sugar stays up and things, and he'll take care of it." I thought this was great, I was reassured. I didn't know what was going on. I didn't know much about these symptoms. I didn't know where they're coming from or what the exact type of workup or evaluation should be initiated. I had just come out of residency, and I knew OBGyn protocols, but for these type of symptoms I was trained to refer a person to their Family Doctor. So the fact that she went there made me reassured. She didn't complain about them anymore after that, that I remember. That also made me feel like, 'okay, this guy's taking care of her.'

Well, several months went by and I remember she was on vacation and she called me one night and said, "Geoff, I have a horrible headache." I'm like, "Mom, what do you mean?" And she said, "Well, I just, I just started having headaches and they feel like the worst headache of my life. I am having one right now, it is so bad that I just can't do anything." she goes, "what do you think?" I said, "Mom, I don't really like that because you're 58 years old, you shouldn't be having new onset headaches at 58 years old. I think you really need to get checked out." She was not in my town so I said, "Mom, I want you to call the doctor and tell your doctor that I am asking for a CT scan or MRI of the brain, because these are not normal. You should not begin having severe headaches at 58 years old. So I want to make sure everything's okay and see if there's anything else going on." She said, "okay." So when she got back from vacation a few days later, she went to her doctor and had a CT scan. I remember that after her CT scan was performed, I was in my private office seeing patients. Shortly after her CT Scan was performed, I got a call from a Nurse Practitioner at the doctor's office where my Mom went. The Nurse Practitioner said, "Hi Dr. Cly, my name is so-and-so. I am the nurse practitioner for Dr. so-and-so. He wanted me to give you a call and tell you that we did your Mom's CT scan and the, the results are not good. There multiple large tumors in her brain, she has advanced brain cancer. We want her to get seen right away by our cancer doctor, the oncologist, and to try to figure out what, what these are and what to do for her."

"What!! No! Oh God ...why?" As you can imagine, this news hit me so hard, it was like a never ending nightmare. Although I know what I was just told, I couldn't grasp the severity of what was about to happen. I was in shock and disbelief. At the same time, I knew and suspected that these tumors could be a sign of something else happening somewhere else in her body. I also knew that this was going to change our family's life and Mom's life most of all. I was reluctant to admit this, but I knew there was a chance that my Mom wouldn't be with us for as many years as I had hoped she would be.

I had just lost my dad 2 years earlier. My mom was my rock, she was the only parent I had left. I was determined not to fail her like I felt that I failed my dad. I didn't know exactly what was going on, but I immediately moved into supportive son mode as well as doctor mode. I pushed my emotions aside and focused on Mom and how to get her the best medical care I could find. I lived in a much larger city, Dayton, Ohio, with much more medical resources than the small city in West Virginia she lived in. I immediately started working on trying to get her in to be seen, to do some other testing to find out if these brain tumors were from the brain or did they come from somewhere else in her body, like metastatic cancer. She had a lot of medical tests done and it turned out she had tumors all over her body, they were everywhere! The brain tumors were metastatic cancer from somewhere else. The tumors in the brain were large and there were many of them.

We were able to get her into treatment with the cancer specialists in Dayton. The treatments were intense, often, and started just about 14 days after getting the original CT results and other results back. The next six months Mom went through intense medical cancer treatments, radiation treatments, chemotherapy, and surgeries. Fortunately, some of the treatments were able to be done in her hometown, Charleston, West Virginia. Thank goodness for the help my Mom got from our family. My aunt Jeannie, Mom's younger sister, was able to actually stay with her in West Virginia where she lived during most of the treatments. I was going back and forth as much as possible while still trying to run an OBGyn office practice as part of a group in Dayton, Ohio. We were praying for the best, and supporting her.

It turned out, the tumors were pancreatic cancer that had metastasized to her brain from the pancreas. Mom was a very spiritual woman and she went through the treatments and all of the radiation with courage. I know she stayed strong for us, her children, and her family. At times during these six months she had moments she wanted to give in, that is for sure, but she continued to fight the cancer. Her courage and bravery were amazingly strong through it all.

Unfortunately, despite all the prayers we sent out, and all the treatments she endured, the cancer kept spreading and getting worse. Eventually, there was no hope left to beat it. I believe she realized it before we did, and she was placed in a home hospice program and all the treatments were stopped. At the time, I didn't understand or accept God's plan for her life. But... she did. Looking back, now I can see how her faith and spirituality were increasing and becoming stronger, even though her body was becoming weaker and being taken over by the cancer.

The weekend after her original diagnosis, I asked my brother, Tony, my sister, Jeanne, our kids, and families as well as my aunts and uncles to come to West Virginia to be with Mom, take pictures, and spend the weekend with her. I wanted all of us to have time and photos with Mom where she was smiling and still looked like our Mom. To be honest, I didn't tell everyone the entire truth about why we were gathering together. Mostly it was to support Mom, and pray, and have some good times with her before the cancer and radiation journey started. But, the part I didn't tell everyone was that I knew she would lose all her hair, and a lot of weight; I knew she may never look the same again, and I knew, deep down, something I didn't even want to think about. She was going to die.

On October 10, 2002, after only 6 months from the original CT scan diagnosis, my Mom died. We only had 6 months from the day of that phone call about her CT scan results. And not 6 months of good times either. It was six months of grueling, heartbreaking, gut wrenching, emotional turmoil for me and our family watching Mom go through exhausting, painful, exasperating cancer treatments that in the end made absolutely no difference and only put her through a living hell.

"Why?!! Why God?...What the f@*k!" I was so angry at God, I was so angry at the world, but really, I was so angry at myself. I had failed my Mom and my Dad. And now they were dead......What kind of a messed up, stupid doctor must I have been if I couldn't even save my Mom or my Dad.....

In 20 years since Mom died, I have only shared those details and emotions and entire story with a handful of people. Most of my family members do not know how I felt on the inside, or the details I shared with you. As I sit here typing this, remembering these moments, I find myself really struggling. For the past several hours as I put the words together to describe the deaths of my Mom and Dad I am hurting. Even though it has been 20 years since they passed, tonight it feels like it is happening all over again. My keyboard is wet with the tears that have suddenly burst from my eyes. My throat is sore from the uncontrollable sobbing that has just sprang forth out of nowhere. The deep, deep aching, unstoppable pain in my chest that occured when I was told my Dad was dead has come back full force tonight as I relive the deaths of my parents. And that awful moment I went into the bedroom and saw that my Mom was dead, and verified that her frail, thin, post chemotherapy, holocaust like, body had no pulse just came rushing back to me with another episode of uncontrollable sobbing. "Oh God....oh God, I just don't understand....." is what I find myself saying tonight, 20 years later.

Fortunately, this time, I have found God's Grace. I no longer have misplaced anger at God. The spiritual journey for me has been a long one, and probably will be the focus of another book. Although I still question why did it have to happen to my parents and my family, I do believe God's plan for me is to be telling you this, and for the information that follows in this book and for the messages of honesty and truthfulness for women everywhere.

The loss of my Mom was awful, and my feelings of guilt and sadness were quickly replaced by anger after she died. You might be thinking that whole experience was awful enough and this journey has to get better, I know that is what I was hoping and praying for as well. But, there is a twist in this story. The next part of this story is a huge part of the journey to creating HonestOBGyn.com and why I stand up for women.

What I found out after Mom passed was that her family doctor had completely and terribly disregarded my Mom. About a year prior to the CT scan, when I asked my Mom to go see her Family Doctor, the one who she went to see when she had these electrical sensations, these buzzing sounds, these flashing lights – he said that she was crazy and she was making this symptoms up and he gave her a diagnosis of psychosomatic, which means the person is making up these symptoms and it's all in their head.

While she was alive I never knew this. This is the same guy who didn't have the decency to call me and tell me as a fellow physician that, 'I'm so sorry', or 'your Mom has tumors in her brain.' He never contacted me, or any of our family, only the nurse practitioner did. That was devastating to find that out. Not only was it devastating to lose my dad and have the doctors treat him the way they did. But then, about two years later, my Mom was blown off by a doctor and wrote down that she was crazy but made her think that he was helping her and caring for her.

The other devastating part is that this was a colleague or a fellow physician that I had placed my trust in who completely disregarded that trust and professionalism. And he not only didn't do what was right, didn't listen to my Mom, didn't think about what was happening, but just wrote her off as crazy and gave her some sugar pills and sent her on her way. If he would have taken the time and done what was right and evaluated her symptoms and said, maybe let's do a CT scan a year ago, it would have allowed her to be with us longer. His carelessness did not allow her to have more time. She didn't even get to know her grandchildren before she died. Even with pancreatic cancer, she still would have left us early, but she would've had so much more time with her family as well.

After this knowledge came out, we wanted to sue and really make this guy pay for what he had done. We had attorneys evaluate the case and the attorneys came back and said, 'really, you could sue. But, because she had pancreatic cancer, the end result probably won't be worth the outcome with a lot of time and energy and money negativity going into this lawsuit where in the end, if she would have only got a few years at best longer. So we ended up saying, you know what, we don't think our Mom would want that. We knew she was such a positive, uplifting person that she wouldn't want us just to be angry and, and hateful and just go into this negative lawsuit. So with that knowledge, we just agreed to move forward with our lives and drop the idea of a lawsuit and just try to live life to the fullest.

That changed my outlook on life because here I had lost both my parents in a very short time. I was the oldest of three kids. I was 32 at the time and had a couple young children. I realized that things can change at any moment. On one hand, I changed my outlook on life and I said, do you know what? I don't know how long I've got but I'm going to try and live it to the fullest. Not that I wasn't living to the fullest. I've always tried to enjoy life and do the most I can do and I have a ton of energy, but this made me realize that I can't wait until retirement for big things to happen or to check off my bucket list. I've got to make sure that I always live to live life to the fullest, enjoy it now, and still plan for retirement later in life. Just in case I don't make it. I want to be able to say that I lived a full life. So that's how I live my life. I'd try to be thankful for every day and live every day to its fullest. I look forward to another day on this earth, but I know that it's ultimately not up to me. Ultimately I really have no control over what happens. I can only enjoy life and people and and serve and give as much as I can while I'm here on a different level.

On the other side of this was a solidification and unfortunate realization that there are significantly more doctors who are bad doctors who make bad decisions and who don't care about their patients. I realized there are a ton more people suffering because of this. To me this was unacceptable. Here, I've worked so hard to become a doctor. I've spent so much time and energy in learning and school and training. I've missed tons of fun times because I was studying so hard all these years at college. I value being a doctor, I'm honored by the trust people place in me and I am so grateful for that trust. To have other fellow colleagues just throw that away, and by their inconsiderate, selfish, and inhuman actions they harm, kill, and injure people, and most of all MY parents! My Mom and Dad had THE worst outcome - wrongful death due to negligence and malpractice.

This ordeal changed my outlook on doctors and medicine. I realized that I have to stand up for the patients. I cannot trust what another doctor says just because they're a doctor. I have to verify things myself, of course it also depends on the severity and difficulty of the situation. If I feel like there is something that is not right or a doctor is doing something that they shouldn't, or a doctor's not taking adequate care of a patient that I'm involved with, I'm going to speak out and I'm going to do what I gotta do to protect that patient. I am going to make sure that that patient heals in the best way possible - THAT became my mission!

Someone told me a long time ago, one of the physicians who trained me, Dr. Ezenagu, he was an upperclassman in my OBGyn residency program. He told me this famous quote, "Trust, but verify". That's something that I've brought into my professional life. Because, if I get a diagnosis from another doctor, then I'll trust that in the sense of, okay, let's work with it and that's our working diagnosis, but I'm going to need to verify that. That quote has made a difference. There are many times in my career where I've found the things that other doctors just blew off, or things that weren't correct. My journey and that quote has completely shaped the way I practice medicine. There have been many patients who have been helped because of my need to trust but verify. I take great pride and honor in being able to make a difference in someone's life. The times I am able to correct an error or find someone's problem when other doctors can't or won't even try happens much too often. These times actually frustrate me because I know that these other doctors could have found the same thing I did and they should have invested the time and care and concern for their patients. One of the largest and most significant examples of this in with my journey into the world of DaVinci robotic laparoscopic surgery that began in 2005.

3 Young Dr. Cly & His Robot named DaVinci

In 2005 I came across a $2.5 million dollar surgical robot that was inside of a closet of the surgery department where I used to work. This thing was collecting dust and not being used by the Heart Surgeons who asked the hospital to buy it. Instantly I recognized this device was the DaVinci Robotic Surgical system. Years earlier I had seen one of the only 2 DaVinci Surgical prototypes in the world when I was training on surgical laparoscopic instruments in Cincinnati, Ohio. At that time I was told it was a new robotic surgery instrument for the heart surgeons. I thought, wow that is cool, but a regular gynecologist like me will never be able to use something like that. Little did I know that in less than 10 years from that moment I would become one of the first Gynecologists in America to use DaVinci, then be a DaVinci champion, and eventually teach most of the gynecologists in my region how to do surgery with it.

Why was this amazing DaVinci robot collecting dust? Well, the heart surgeons did a few cases on it and didn't like it at all and they just put it in the closet where it was collecting dust. In addition to the $2.5 million dollar cost, the hospital also had to pay for a $250,000 yearly maintenance contract on it. Immediately I thought, wow, I can use this thing for Gynecology surgery. I had performed hundreds of laparoscopies without the DaVinci, but I realized that this would allow me to do amazing things for my patients. The DaVinci would allow me to do complex gynecology surgeries on women through dime size incisions and not have to cut women open any longer with a large, 6 inch or 10 inch painful incision. This was the true game changer for patients. Not only could women go home the same day and drive the next day, they would have minimal pain and less complications, less bleeding, and most importantly they could get their lives back with significantly less recovery time. For example, back to work in a little as 1 week compared to 6 weeks. Driving the next day instead of 2 weeks. Minimal pain or no pain compared to the pain of a cesarean section type of surgery.

I realized this was absolutely in the best interest of my patients and I dedicated myself to learning how to use it, now matter how much more difficult or scary it would be for me. I knew it was the right thing to do. Interestingly, this same thing with heart surgeons hating this system and putting it in closets was happening all over the country. So as a result, those of us gynecologists with a DaVinci system at our disposal began to collaborate and help each other learn and adapt our surgeries. The reason this was important in my journey is because I got to train with and be trained by the best DaVinci gynecologists in the entire world. The best and first leader was Arnie Advincula, MD, he was in Michigan and hosted the 1st Annual World Robotics Gynecology Conference. He had performed the most DaVinci cases in the entire world and still to this day is considered the Guru. I remember going to that conference and there were only about 50 or so Gynecologists attending. Now the DaVinci conferences have thousands of doctors attending and learning.

In late 2005, I was the only gynecologist in my city, Fort Wayne, Indiana, doing DaVinci robotic surgery. I was the first one in the Northeast Indiana region. And I was the only one for three years doing DaVinci robotic gynecology cases in Fort Wayne, Indiana. What the DaVinci allowed for is that women who would have had to be cut open, no longer needed to be. They could have small incisions but have big surgeries like complex hysterectomies or prolapse surgeries or endometriosis resections performed through these small incisions. And then they could go home the same day or next day with very little pain - this was revolutionary and amazing.

I get into specifics about DaVinci and in the upcoming chapters. But the next thing I am going to tell you about was the beginning of a new era and it was about time as well. What started happening was that I would have patients come to me, and they were new patients to me, but they had been seen by other doctors in my town. They had heard about the DaVinci system and they wanted to have a DaVinci hysterectomy. One particular patient came to me and she was an author, a business owner and an entrepreneur. She was in her sixties, a wonderful lady. She said that she wanted the DaVinci procedure. She was a perfect candidate for the DaVinci. She did not want to be cut open, and without the DaVinci she would have had to have an abdominal hysterectomy (which she refused). So she told her doctor, who happened to be a woman doctor here in town, "I want the DaVinci." Her doctor flat out told her that she cannot have the DaVinci, that she was not a candidate for the DaVinci. She instead recommended an open abdominal hysterectomy.

When she came to me with this information I was at first somewhat perplexed and I told the lady, I said, well, you're actually the perfect candidate for DaVinci surgery. All of these reasons, that are going on with you and for your desires and your goals, DaVinci surgery is actually the perfect fit for you. I said I'm not sure what the other doctor was saying, but I did know that the other female doctor in town did not do DaVinci's. She only did the old fashioned hysterectomies. And so I said, look, I think you are a candidate. I'm willing to schedule you for a DaVinci but if I'm missing something, we're going to find it out during surgery. But, I cannot find a reason why you are not a candidate and you should not have the DaVinci. You're actually the perfect candidate.

I scheduled the surgery for her and she agreed to have the procedure. She did great, had the DaVinci hysterectomy, got back to work within the week. She had minimal pain and was driving right away.

The reason I bring the story up is because that was the first time in my town, I realized that there was a doctor flat out lying to her patients because that doctor did not want to lose money or lose business. The interesting thing with this is that scenario continued to happen several more times with that same doctor. The patients found out about me would come over to me and tell me that the doctor said the same thing. I would tell the patients, "Here's what I'm finding, here's what I recommend, and you have to decide what you would like to do." I usually would be asked to do the surgery and the patients did great, because they were good candidates. After three years that doctor who was lying to her patients finally decided to learn how to do DaVinci surgeries and she became an excellent DaVinci doctor and did almost everything with the DaVinci. This was when I realized that the patients choices are going to change the physician's behavior. So by patients demanding they want this newer procedure, they're not going to tolerate the older painful outdated surgery that causes them more pain, more time off work, and more complications. The simple truth is that the patients are the key to changing a doctor's behavior by how their decisions affect the finances of the doctor and whether that doctor is getting enough business or not.

I bring that story up because on this journey of being a physician, in all the nonsense that happened with the other physicians, I quickly realized, okay, I'm going to continue to do this. It is right for patients and even though I've been made fun of in the doctor's lounges for years for doing this I am not going to stop. I knew it was the right thing to do. I realized that the patients would drive the business. After three years, other competing doctors in town started to want to learn how to do DaVinci surgeries. So I decided to train other doctors and to teach them because if, if I could teach them the skills, then I was sure they would see the light like I did.

Over these early years I got a reputation as the most skilled DaVinci gynecologist in Northeast Indiana, simply because no one else was doing it for three years and I had a huge lead in the amount of DaVinci experience. I was doing them as much as appropriately possible and people started to come requesting that I do the surgery for them. I also realized that this is something I've loved to do. I was passionate about it. I liked teaching other doctors. I liked to do the surgeries. I love it when patients recover so well and so fast.

One of the early cases that I did that also told me this was a technology that was going to continue to change the face of medicine. In the beginning, I actually had women asking to be my first case, they trusted me. (For this I was/am grateful and thankful for their trust). In my first case, I did a hysterectomy on a patient who was over 300 pounds. Without the DaVinci technology, this lady would have had to have been opened up with a very large incision because of how much she weighed. She had a lot of fatty tissue on her abdomen. Because of that, I would have to make a wider incision because of the depth to get to the uterus going through all the fatty tissue and through the muscles is deeper. So when we make a bigger incision to get more access on a person who's obese or over 300 pounds, that increases the pain. It increases the risk of healing problems. It increases the risk of infection, increases the risk of bleeding. In those patients, without getting too technical are not candidates for vaginal hysterectomy, or for the regular non DaVinci laparoscopic hysterectomy because of those same reasons related to access and depth of the incision. Having this DaVinci technology allowed me to do a small incision minimally invasive hysterectomy on this lady who was over 300 pounds.

Liz (whose name was changed for privacy), one of my first cases, knew I was new at this and she was still agreeable to let me do the procedure. In patients who are obese, when they have a abdominal hysterectomy, they're in a lot of pain and many times they're in the hospital for two or three days. Just trying to walk is extremely painful, they can't drive for two weeks, and go back to work for six weeks. It's a rough situation for someone who's obese and they're at a big risk for a wound infection, which means that that whole incision has a higher chance to get infected and then it's opened up to drain the infection and in those cases it takes months to heal. It can be a nightmare.

So I did this case, it took me three hours. It was one of my first cases. It was way back before we had some of the high tech, newer instruments and adapters that make the surgeries go so much faster nowadays. However, it was successful. The surgery went fine other than taking a long time. And the next day I went into round on her to see how she was doing. What happened next was another, "Eureka!" moment and I knew this technology is going to change the world.

So I got to the hospital around nine o'clock. I think I told her I was going to be there a little bit earlier. When I got in a room at nine o'clock in the morning, the morning after her surgery, she was dressed sitting on the side of her bed and angry because I was late and she wanted to go home! When she got mad at me, I realized that she had no idea how amazing she's feeling compared to what would have happened with the old fashioned way. I was excited because here's a lady who should, who should not have been feeling this good. If she had had any one of the other doctors in the town do a surgery for her, she would would be in bed in pain and barely able to move at this moment. So her super fast recovery told me that this is the way, this is the future and there's no going back! I knew this is what I had to continue to do so because it was right for patients. This was back in 2005. At this time, I had not yet thought of the website, HonestOBGyn.com or that I would ever be writing a book. But I knew that I wanted to continue with this amazing DaVinci technology and teach as many people as I could.

In the early years, as a young doctor performing surgeries with a brand new technology called the DaVinci system, I was being made fun of by OBGyn colleagues. I was using this machine that was developed by the military and cost about $2.5 million dollars. Remember, at this time only a handful of us around the country were doing DaVinci surgery as far as gynecologists go. Also remember that originally, the first uses of it were for heart surgeons to be able to do DaVinci heart surgery, which is much easier for patients. And many hospitals around the country bought DaVinci systems for the heart surgeons to do these heart surgery, DaVinci cases. What happened all over the country was the heart surgeons hated the machine. Heart surgeons in general back in those days like to crack a chest. They like to feel the beating heart. They like to work directly on the heart. And at the same time, all of them wanted to have the latest technology. Heart surgery brings in a lot of revenue for hospitals. The hospitals around the country bought these machines for the heart surgeons and that happened here in this town. The hospital I was working at bought the machine for the heart surgeon. They had a big media splash, I think they did a case or two and they hated it and they put it in a closet. So the DaVinci system that cost $2.5 million dollars with a $250,000 dollar service contract or warranty program per year was sitting in the closet collecting dust.

I immediately realized I could use this machine. I can figure out something to do with it. And so I contacted the DaVinci representative and started the whole process that changed my life. What I became known for and good at, was DaVinci gynecologic surgery. The hospital liked it because now they have an expensive asset that is no longer collecting dust and it's gonna be able to generate revenue. I was happy because I knew it was great for patients and it would be a game changer. Also this, it's important to know, that I did not get paid anymore money for using this machine. Actually, we get paid more money for doing an open hysterectomy than we did when we do doing a DaVinci system or vaginal hysterectomy. An open large incision hysterectomy only takes about 30 minutes and a DaVinci is about 1.5 hours. So I was getting paid less money per case and could not do as many cases per day either.

I was in the lounge one day and one of my OBGyn colleagues came in who was a very busy OBGyn here in town and very popular. And he said: "Geoff, you know ... I can do three abdominal hysterectomies at the same time it takes you to do one DaVinci hysterectomy. And I make three times the amount of money, and, at six weeks post-op our patients are the same! At six weeks my patients can drive back to work and they feel normal again." And I said to him: "Man, you're missing the point! It's not about the six weeks! They can go home the next day. They don't have pain. They feel good. They drive the next day. It's not about the money, it's about the patients!"

For three years, that's what many of the doctors in my town did to me. They just kind of made fun of me and snickered at me. And they were reveling in the fact that they were making more money and they were doing more surgeries faster than me. And then there's this crazy guy Cly, operating this crazy machine that takes more time. It took about two hours. It still takes probably about two hours on average. Maybe - maybe - an hour and a half on a straight forward hysterectomy case. But, the large outdated abdominal hysterectomy, the doctor can be done 30 minutes or 45 minutes and get paid more money. And so for three years I was the comic relief for many doctors in town here, but the patients are what kept me going and gave me strength. Because I continued to see my patients heal great, feel great, and get back to the life they love quickly.. They felt great. It was just amazing how wonderful they felt and that is what kept me going and keeps me going now. It's because I want to help people and I want to do what's right.

Interestingly enough: again, the same thing happened with this doctor as did with the female doctor. As I mentioned to you, this doctor said one day that he wanted to get trained because he was losing patients. Women were leaving the other doctors because they didn't want to be cut open anymore. They wanted to have the best treatment option.

And so at the 3 year point, doctors started asking and wanting to get trained on the DaVinci system. When other doctors in town started wanting to be trained to do DaVinci surgeries, it was like a huge domino effect. Once, a couple of them said, yeah, they wanted to do it,..... and then boom! Everybody else in town wanted to learn, almost everybody else wants to learn because nobody wants to be left out. There were still a few holdouts, but I would say about 80% of doctors in Fort Wayne started to learn the DaVinci and around 2008, 2009.

So, who should train my competitors? Well, I volunteered to be the Doctor who trained them. Why you might ask? At the time, one of my mentors, Dr. Thomas Payne, the first private OBGyn who did 200 surgeries and a case study proving how well DaVinci is for private practice as well as academic University hospitals, and one of the really great OBGyn DaVinci doctors who trained me, gave me some wise insight. I called him and talked to him and I said: "Hey, these guys in town want to get trained. They're my competition. What do you think?" He said: "Geoff, either you could train them and become their mentor or you could block them and not train them, but they're going to bring in someone else from another area to train. Just like I used to go out and train docs outside of this town and other areas of the country." I said: "Yep, that makes total sense." So I offered to train as many people as I could in town and teach them the best skills that I knew and the tricks that I learned over the three years. It actually brought many of us closer together and we became better colleagues friends and developed amicable trust. That being said, we were still competitors, but now patients referred to me as, "The DaVinci doctor who teaches doctors how to do surgery" and fortunately that skyrocketed my credibility and patients continued to ask me to do their surgeries.

Training more doctors on DaVinci was a very positive thing and allowed more patients to get the best treatment possible. And once again, the patients, drove the business because they were demanding to have the best treatments possible. They didn't want the old way anymore. And they had heard about it by word of mouth they'd heard about it by the commercials. And so that was about 2008, 2009 and I continued to help train docs and continue to do so. And now almost all OBGyn in this town use the Da Vinci system.

However, there are still a couple of doctors in this town who, even though the DaVinci system has been out for 15 years, who are still refusing to learn the DaVinci system AND still do outdated abdominal hysterectomies with large painful incisions on their patients. Fairly recently, one of my former partners, now a former friend, said to me, "Geoff, I'm 10 years away from retirement. I don't want to learn how to do the DaVinci and I'm going to do it the old way. It's just fine. And that's the way it is." I told him, you're missing the point and this is another one of the moments that made me realize patients are still being lied to and they're still being misled and they're still not being told the truth. These doctors are not telling them the truth or informing them with all their options. Why? Because if the patient leaves and has the surgery done somewhere else, the doctor loses money. Doctors cannot get a referral fee for referring you to another doctor. It's illegal. And so if a doctor chooses not to learn the DaVinci, which has been out for 15 years and they lose a patient, they lose money.

Interestingly enough around 2017, the same doctor who told me he wasn't going to learn DaVinci, was doing a surgery in operating room 1 and I was doing a DaVinci hysterectomy in operating room 2. I didn't know what he was doing. He didn't know what I was doing because we don't know what each other's doing due to HIPPA privacy laws. We might talk in the lounge sometimes, but many times we don't even see each other until after the surgery. So that was on a Friday morning, several ago. I was on call on Saturday, So I had to go see the patients in the hospital, discharge them, make sure they're okay. And my patient had gone home already because of the DaVinci. And so his patient had the old fashioned hysterectomy. And because I was rounding on her, I had to look at her chart and see what was going on with her and take care of her.

What I saw was frustrating, and was disheartening and also made me angry. And that was because when I looked at her chart and saw the reason she had the hysterectomy and saw her notes about her uterus and saw the ultrasound, it was crystal clear to me that she had been lied to. She was told she was not a candidate for the DaVinci based on his notes that said she was not a candidate and he did her surgery the old fashioned way with a large painful incision. She was in the hospital for two more days, couldn't drive for two weeks, a lot more pain, and off work for six weeks. Only because he doesn't want to learn how to do the DaVinci system. This patient had not been told the truth. This patient had no idea that she could have had the DaVinci done by one of the other eight partners in the office and there were only about two to three docs at that time who had chosen not to do the DaVinci system.

This particular doc misled his patient. I was able to see it firsthand and I felt guilty because here I am rounding on her. I didn't want to rub salt in the wound and say, Oh man, if only you'd have the DaVinci, you'd be home right now like my patient is. So I just tried to make her feel the best she could. I tried to make sure her pain was minimal and I think I discharged her on Sunday, the next second day. This really did hurt me inside because this was my colleague. Here I'm trying to do the best I can do for patients and this patient didn't even know other options and she didn't know her doctor misled her.

Now, this information can never be revealed for the most part because of the privacy laws. And that's how these doctors get away with stuff is because the privacy laws prevent other people from looking into the exact details if there are no complications. The medical system still states a doctor can choose the route of hysterectomy or surgery based on their own experience, which is also very frustrating to me. If you don't know how to do to Da Vinci and your experience is the old fashioned way, the system says that's still okay for you to do an outdated surgery. But to me it isn't. It's the same thing in many ways to me as if you go to a car lot and you're looking to buy a new car and you see two cars sitting next to each other. They both look the same on the outside. When you test drive one of them, it doesn't have air condition and it has a roll of windows, but the salesman doesn't tell you that the car right next to it is air conditioned. It has roll up windows and it's the same price. The salesman is trying to steer you into buying the car that has lesser options because the salesman wants to make, make a profit off that sale. That to me is, is very similar to what's happening in medicine in this arena.

There is a name for it, it's called "DaVinci bait and switch". The DaVinci reps came up with this name. Here is how it works: some doctors will go learn how to do the DaVinci system. They'll go to the three or four day course, which is paid for by the hospital usually. And then they'll get a certificate. After that they never or rarely use the DaVinci. And they bait and switch. They advertise to their patients that they're robotic DaVinci gynecologic surgeons. Then when the patient comes in for a consultation, they tell the patient, "Oh, well you're not a candidate for the DaVinci. So I'm going to do it the old way." Then they stack the outdated abdominal hysterectomy cases and they bust out a ton of cases on a day. They make three or four times the amount of money. And then patient never knows, she was actually misled, baited and switched and lied to and could have had a better treatment, a better surgery for the same price that she paid for the other one.

Quickly, I want to tell you something that is very important and non-DaVinci doctors need to hear what I am about to say. If you don't have a daVinci in your town, then either offer your patient a laparoscopic or vaginal surgery and if that is not possible, then be honest and tell her where the closest daVinci is and allow her to choose what surgery she wants to undergo. If the patient wants to have an old fashioned hysterectomy that is acceptable and you have informed her truthfully.

Also, there are many OBGyns who are not DaVinci trained that WILL do the right thing and refer their patients somewhere that has a DaVinci or give them a minimally invasive surgery instead of baiting and switching.

When these events happened several years ago it solidified in my mind that I had to reach out beyond my office walls. It is time to tell women the truth and to make sure they know their up to date surgical and treatment options. I want to make sure they have honest OBGyn information.

Women deserve to have a voice and be empowered with knowledge so that if someone's trying to bait and switch them or someone's trying to minimize them or patronize them or offer them an outdated procedure, they now can say, "Wait, don't take my uterus." I want the better option. I want the nonsurgical option. I don't want to be cut open anymore. I now have the knowledge to tell you, Dr. Oldfashioned, that I'm not going to accept that.

4 Getting Fired for HonestOBGyn.com

Those events all led to me saying, "I'm going to create a website to tell people the truth anywhere in the country." Actually I wanted it to be anywhere in the world, but my attorney said, you have to focus on only America since you're an American doctor. Okay, that's fine for now.... But I'm still gonna keep trying to tell everyone the truth. So that's what led to HonestOBGyn.com being created. And it has taken a while to create it. My team and I are still building on to the site and adding more pieces all the time. The goals of this journey are to help women, in all aspects of health.

Several years ago when my wife Megan, was pregnant with our son Christian, we were both learning different business aspects, leadership skills, and taking personal development courses that would teach us and allow us to spread our message with a new website type of business. We realized that the message was truth and honesty in the world of medicine, specifically obstetrics and gynecology. My wife, Megan, was a labor and delivery nurse and me being an OBGyn, we had expertise in the area of women's health and labor and delivery. And so late in 2015 when she was pregnant with our son Christian, we both made a decision to move forward and create a website called HonestOBGyn.com to spread honesty and transparency so women can get up to date and accurate treatment information regardless of where they lived. We wanted them to be empowered with the knowledge to guide them to live their best life and getting back to taking care of their family and being healthy again.

We thought of it much like a GPS in the way that when I am in a taxi cab, many times I will pull up my GPS in the back seat just to make sure that the taxi cab driver is heading in the right direction and most accurate direction to get me to my destination. So that was the thought, how can we give women the information they need to help them get the treatment they need. So we decided to create HonestOBGyn.com and we partnered with a web company. We hired some attorneys and worked with some branding and marketing specialist to help us create the site as well as a business that would accomplish these goals.

This project has taken a while because we wanted it to be thorough and then as we got into it, we realized that there were many more pieces of this website that would be important and necessary. One of them being some type of downloadable printed pocket guide or comprehensive guide that women could print off, read through and take it to their doctor to give to the doctor and say, " Doctor, here's what I heard about on the internet, can you tell me more about these treatments." We also wanted women to be able to search on the internet and find our website so that in addition to going to popular websites like WebMD, they would also find HonestOBGyn.com and no matter whether it was day or night or weekends, they could get the information they need.

Also, as I found in my practice, I would often see women and tell them that based on what I'm finding, they need a surgery or even a hysterectomy in some cases. Later they would go home and tell their partner, but their partners really didn't have the same level of understanding because their partner was not there for the visit. So I also wanted a way that men or women could look this information up and find out the honest, truthful information about these procedures in alternatives, as well as verify that the doctor they talked to, no matter where their doctor was in the country, was guiding them in the right direction.

This type of specific, directed, physician level OB or GYN treatment information is not available to the normal public. It's available to us as doctors, or us as nurses, because we have a medical reference books that educate us and guide us on the treatment recommendations. And so I know as a doctor that if a woman is diagnosed with uterine fibroids for example, then these are the steps that we as doctors have to follow to evaluate the problem, diagnose the problem and the treatments we are supposed to recommend and in the step by step order we're supposed to recommend them.

I knew that giving this type of specific physician level information to women would create an even playing field for them no matter where they are at in the country. And so if a woman is being told one thing that's different than another woman in another area of the country, they would now know the truth and they could hand this information to their doctor. And say, 'wait a second doctor, before you cut me open, please tell me about these alternative procedures that HonestOBGyn and Dr. Cly are mentioning here on this piece of paper.'

I also realized that there is a lot of value in educational seminars. I've done educational seminars and TV shows for the last 16 years and I wanted to be able to offer that to women or their partners anytime, 24/7 as well. And so along with the downloadable pocket guides, I created educational seminars on each specific topic so that women could not only download the guide, but they could also watch me talking to them in an educational seminar just like I've done on TV, just like I've done it for public events in my local town.

This way it could be reproduced and recorded and played at anytime, 24/7, so that women from all over the country could get that same type of educational seminar. I also realized that there's going to be women who want to talk with me personally and ask questions. And so I created an aspect of the site that allows women to access me in a private Facebook group where I would be able to answer their questions 24/7. In addition to just posting questions, I wanted to offer live Facebook or live video events where I could give them an educational seminar and then they can personally ask questions. Just like I was doing a seminar in a local town or a local meeting room that I've done many times before. Even on the TV live shows I've done the same thing where I talk about a topic and at the end of the show I do live TV questions and answers.

Well, one other aspect that we knew would happen was that doctors would try to claim that what I'm saying is wrong or disagree with what I'm saying. And as I have seen personally in my local town, there are doctors who have lied to women about the different procedures because those doctors decided not to learn the procedures and they don't want to lose those clients or the money that they would get from those surgeries. So when this happens I want the women or their partners to have another option and to know that there are doctors in their local town who are doing up to date treatments and who have learned the latest type of surgeries, like the daVinci surgery. That other aspect of the website is a physician directory where a person can put in their zip code and they can find a daVinci surgeon in their zip code anywhere in the country. This is something that is free and important so a woman or partner doesn't feel like they have no other options if their doctor flat out refuses to acknowledge some of these other treatments or alternatives that would otherwise be the appropriate fit for particular people.

We began the journey on the website by creating several businesses to would comply with all the legal connections and behind the scenes interactions, laws, and rules, because I am a physician and there are certain rules for a business in this type of area. Also, I had to follow the rules of my employment contract with my employer so that I wouldn't cause any issues in that arena as well. From the beginning we had a total of five attorneys helping us with this project and there were a lot of complexities that I learned about along the way.

One of the things the attorneys told me in the beginning was that there is a law called the Federal Civil Monetary Penalties Act. Which states that patients cannot be given gifts or things that could be construed as gifts because that would violate that federal law and it would be very much like enticing patients with gifts to come to me as a doctor. Originally, I had thought that any patient who comes to the office to see me would get this information during their visit and when they check out they could have this kind of written treatment plan as well.

My attorney said that actually my office patients must be kept separate from any client on the web who downloads this information or pays for the private Facebook group, or other educational videos because it would violate that federal law. That was something we learned and we certainly did not want to violate any rules or laws, so we realized early on that the website, HonestOBGyn.com, would need to be kept completely separate from the medical practice and any of my medical patients.

Another thing I had not realized was that in the contract of my former employer, it stated that anything I created with another colleague would be considered the intellectual property of my employer. What that means is that if I asked any of my other OBGyn colleagues to participate in developing one of the pocket guides or one of the educational videos, and because we both work at that hospital, what we created would technically be the intellectual property of the hospital. The attorneys said that I had to create these things on my own, otherwise it would violate the contract.

That actually made the whole journey take a lot longer, because in the beginning I had thought about talking with some of my colleagues and we could do this together and create these pocket guides and treatment plans. But because of the contractual rules in my employment contract, I realized I had to do this on my own. I spent many nights and weekends when Megan was pregnant with Christian, and then our last baby, Victoria, trying to come up with these things and create these pocket guides and do the research, and do the background information to make sure that the information was accurate.

Something else the attorney pointed out was that anything I created had to be done off the employer or hospital's property and it could not be created on their equipment. What that means is that whenever I worked on a laptop to write these pocket guides or do the research, I had to do it on my own laptop, it couldn't be a laptop that was owned by the hospital. And since all of us physicians are given a loaner laptop to use, I had to go out and purchase my own laptop for the business, and that to be done completely separately.

That was okay, but that was another piece to this process. Additionally, I couldn't work on the site when I was at the property of the hospital or former employer because the same thing, everything would be considered their intellectual property if I was creating these new educational things when I was on their property. Fortunately, I found an amazing coworking entrepreneur office space downtown Fort Wayne, The Atrium. It was there where I rented a desk and I have my original website office. I would go after work in the evening while Megan was pregnant with Christian and then Victoria and spend a few hours there many many nights for much of her pregnancies and create this information using the computer that I purchased separately in the office space that I purchased separately.

I knew that I had a limited amount of time in the sense of once the babies were born, I figured things would get more hectic of course, and so I wanted to be home with them and helping Megan and with the other kids as well. Even though I was trying to get everything finished by the time they were born, working on it by myself in the evenings just didn't provide enough time because I still was an OB-GYN during the day and seeing patients and doing surgeries at the former hospital where I'd been for 16 years in total.

Around this time, my former office nurse, Megan U, (yes, a different Megan than my wife), announced she was leaving the office and going to work at the hospital. Megan U and I had worked together for about 10 years and she was the one who had scheduled my surgeries, rounded on patients in the hospital after surgery and gave pre-op instructions, among many other things. Since she was going to be working less at the hospital I asked her if I could hire her on the side to help me with some background research for the pocket guides and help with future social media posts and administrative things for the website. I knew she was loved by my patients and I trusted her which was very important from my standpoint. She agreed and during the preparation, she would gather the background research on treatment protocols that helped me put stuff together. But most importantly, her assistance allowed me to spend more time at home with the babies, Christian and Victoria. Without Megan's help this would have taken a lot longer to create.

The businesses got created in January, 2017, and the original 1st version of the website went live on September 27th, 2017. The original version was a basic website that went up to start getting background links together. I had written the 40+ articles that are still available about different medical and OBGyn subjects, and those were in the background trying to establish links to get a higher status in the Google searches. After those were done, then I continued to create more of these modules and pocket guides but it took a lot of time. Ultimately, the final aspects of the website in its final form, where it could be launched with the media release and the press releases wasn't ready until April of 2019.

Now during this time, as I was embarking on this project, my wife Megan, was helping me and even though she was at home taking care of the kids, I would be bouncing things off of her all the time. She would give me guidance, give me recommendations,and was my sounding board and my strength to help me continue to move forward with the website. During this same time I was learning about marketing, branding, and web design.

I had to learn the behind the scenes aspects of the business. We partnered with Gerry Foster for the branding aspect and to hone the message. Gerry Foster is a fantastic branding expert, he actually is the branding expert for Stedman Graham, Oprah Winfrey's partner. He was one of the branding experts way back, who came up with the "ring around the collar" slogan for one of the laundry detergents.

That journey learning with him was kind of a process where I had to learn about branding and then develop the HonestOBGyn message. Gerry helped me put together what's important and how to communicate it to people on the internet or in the media. He was teaching me how to take my interaction and message in the office that is very personal on a one-on-one level out to a mass media event and still keep it personal. That was a very interesting and worthwhile process. I found it challenging and a different type of skill. In the end, it is the branding that you see today on the website. I recommend him highly and his website is gerryfosterbranding.com

In addition to this, there were so many other aspects happening also. I had a friend of mine who is still a huge business mentor to me today, Michael Silvers. He was one of the leaders who was in a company that Megan and I were learning from,

Success Resources Global. At the time it was called Peak Potentials, and then New Peaks, and then eventually it became Success Resources Global.

Michael Silvers knew about the project and he recommended that I get a business aND personal coach. He guided me to my incredible coach, Brigitta Hoeferle, an amazing woman, an amazing business coach, an excellent personal coach, and a woman with tremendous wisdom and insight. Her business coaching was the main thing that helped me keep this whole project on track, together, and moving forward. Additionally, she helped coach and guide me with the personal challenges that come up during life. Her guidance has been invaluable to me over the last few years. Brigitta helped me focus the things I needed to work on and stay on track to get website launched, get the businesses created, get the behind-the-scenes stuff done, as well as get this book ready to be uploaded to Amazon.

As far as having a personal and a business coach, I have found it invaluable and I know I'm going to continue coaching lifelong. Brigitta has been amazing. If you are interested in learning more, she has a website, nlpatlanta.com. I highly recommend her if you're interested in elevating your life, your business, and yourself to another level. That's what she is excellent at doing.

Along this journey in the last several years, my friend Michael Silvers has helped guide Megan and I to important business conferences and personal development. Along this journey with Michael another huge mentor for me was Adam Markel. Adam is an amazing speaker and an amazing trainer. He helped me with personal development, to elevate myself to a level higher than I ever thought I could be. With his guidance I gained a new level of confidence and outlook on life and realized I could do things that I never thought possible. From a personal level, from a speaking level, from a level of helping to unblock myself with negative thoughts. He taught me how to think bigger and go bigger than ever before.

I wanted to mention Adam Markel, because without his guidance there's no way I would have even been able to start this whole process back in 2017. From 2013 to 2016, Adam Markel's training is what prepared Megan and I for this journey. We both found that his training and his guidance for us in the years leading to HonestOBGyn were amazing and we are so grateful to Adam.

Along these last couple of years in addition to trying to do the website, part of it was learning the branding, learning the marketing, learning the business strategy, learning the sales strategy, learning the different types of media outlets plus the social media ins-and-outs. Interestingly, Michael Silvers is also a part of Powerteam International, which is run by an incredible business man and guru, Bill Walsh, who has taught me so much about the behind-the-scenes aspects of online business, reaching out with social media, how to develop your business speaking skills, and so many other hugely important aspects of business.

What Bill Walsh helped me do is take all the aspects of this website and this business and help accelerate them, moving forward to get things up and running and on track. Currently I'm still learning from Bill Walsh and Powerteam International, and Michael Silvers is part of the mastermind program I am in to continue to turbocharge aspects of business and to fine tune them. Without those people, I would not know how to move forward with several business aspects that come up along the way.

As we're getting close to having the website ready to launch with all the components finalized where they're all kind of connected and put together, I was introduced to my media specialist and press release specialist, Angel Tuccy. Angel is an expert in radio, media press releases, marketing and how to get your message out there. She was instrumental in helping develop and create the press releases that we've sent out, as well as helping me launch the social media aspect of the website back in April and May of 2019.

Angel was introduced to me through Bill Walsh and Powerteam International. I found the skills that these people have is something that I've never seen before. I've always been in the medical profession and I haven't needed to have my own media person or my own press releases, or have my own business with the social media and the marketing aspects from that sense since everything was run through my employer in the past.

So it was with these experts I was able to get my message created and start to send it out to the world. This history I just mentioned brings you up to date on the behind the scenes activity that led up to the shocking events by my former employer that occurred once my first press release was completed.

Everyone wants to know what happened at my former employer and why I suddenly 'was gone". Here is the factual account of those details:

I had been working with attorneys for months, years actually to complete this project, and I had spoken with the CEO of my former employer about six months prior to the website being ready to launch. And I had spoken to my direct supervisor physician around the same time, and I let them know that I was developing a website with medical education aspect and that I was not going to be practicing medicine online, meaning I wasn't going to be seeing patients and taking their information and then assessing them and then prescribing a treatment or planning to do surgeries for them. I was providing education, and the way that I'm doing that is a person already has a diagnosis from their doctor. And based on that diagnosis I'm telling them the treatment options, essentially, the same thing I would do if I was given an educational seminar on fibroids or hysterectomy or abnormal bleeding.

My attorney was communicating with me about the process, and we were trying to follow all of the contractual agreements that were in my employment contract. I had been under the impression that when I was ready for the press release to be sent to the media, that I should let the employer hospital know about it so they can check it and they could edit it, and they could make sure that it was appropriate for them and that I didn't say anything negative or cause any problems for my employer. Around the time we were close to launching, I developed this press release with Angel Tuccy, my media expert. I think the first press release we created was a very good press release.

My attorney checked it and we edited it to make sure that it followed the guidelines and the rules. Then I sent it to my former employer and said, "Hey, I'm launching this website and here's the press release. Please look at it, check it, edit it, let me know what you think. If you can get it back to me soon, I have some interviews lined up for the following week to talk about the website". Well, that's where everything hit the fan, to be quite honest.

What happened next? I got a response from my employer that stated in an email, basically : 'What are you doing? We can't approve this press release until we know about this project and don't have any information about this project/business/website and we need to look into this further.' Well, I was pretty confused. I was under the impression that the attorneys on my side and the attorneys on the hospital side had been communicating for months, ever since I had told the CEO and my supervisor that I was working on this website. They both told me to follow the appropriate rules. And I said, "Okay, that's what I will do."

And so after I sent them the press release, there was this "shotgun surprise" effect that I was confused by. I responded to the email to COO of employer and stated , 'I don't understand. I thought you guys had known about this website and our attorneys have been talking for months now. I'm surprised that you're surprised.'

Essentially my attorney was talking with me and we were talking through attorneys that my employer wanted more information and they had concerns. I tried to answer all those concerns in written form and tried to be as upfront and honest and tell them the same thing as I just told you, for example, about the reasons I created it by myself outside of the office and hospital was so I didn't violate the contract. Or the reason I hadn't talk been talking about it with my colleagues was because it could violate the intellectual property rules and et cetera, et cetera. I was trying to follow the rules, and it was important for me to tell people Honest OBGyn information.

Now it's important to know that I realized when I was creating the website that the website really was meant for people outside of the area where I could see patients. Women who were within the range of my office and the hospital, which was about two hours drive time, would come and see me and in those cases there was no reason for them to go on the website. It made more sense for them to come and see me and have an appointment and get a direct opinion or having me do their surgery or deliver their baby. The goal of the website was to reach people from all over the country who couldn't come and see me or didn't live close enough to come and see me.

I was trying to answer my former employer questions and I was confused and frustrated at the same time that this was becoming such a big deal because I thought everything had been worked out in the background by the attorneys months earlier, especially since I had a total of five attorneys working on this project over the last several years.

One of my former colleagues, former friends, and the person who was also the director of our division came to me and said, essentially, long story short, "Geoff, why can't you just tell women in your office the truth and Honest OBGyn stuff?" And I said, "Well, I do tell people in my office the truth about Honest OBGyn options, and, second, I'm not a doctor for just this hospital. I didn't become a doctor just because of the hospital I work at. I became a doctor to help women and patients no matter where they're at." It was and is very important to me to try to spread the message that I've talked about in this book to anywhere I can so that all women from everywhere had Honest OBGyn information.

And this person was also someone who was practicing differently and did not have DaVinci skills and had chosen at that time not to learn the DaVinci skills. Now, fortunately, he was sending patients who might be a DaVinci case to some of our junior partners, but it was also someone who said, "I don't want to learn how to do DaVinci." And so whether or not this was a factor in what happened over the next couple of days, I'm not sure, but I have to wonder. My attorney said that the hospital was trying to determine what to do, and essentially they had asked me to or requested me to give them the website. And my director told me that if I would give them the website, they would turn it into a hospital website, and I would not be in charge of it, and I would not be able to do media events or talk about it on TV, but it would become a part of the hospital website. I told him that that's not something that I'm comfortable or want to do because I developed this to be something that I could do to reach out to women from all over the country. I also hoped that it would bring in some income so I could pay for the whole project and then put some money away for college for the 6 children that my wife and I have.

Even though, the goal was to charge very low amounts of money for people who are interested in being part of private Members group, it was something that we had spent a lot of money creating and had cost a lot of money over the years to come up with the final product. I wanted to recoup those investments, or at least that was the goal. And at the time when all this activity was occurring at my former employer, this website had not made any money. It was actually in the negative from all the expenses. I had no idea what would happen next. I had hoped that it would do very well, but I certainly wasn't about to just turn it over to the hospital because they demanded it.

My attorney I sent a letter back to the employer with the explanation and the goals of the website. It said something to the effect of; "Here's what I am trying to do. I'm trying to educate women who are not in this area. And that I felt like it was not mutually exclusive, but that the website could help educate women from all over and then I would be able to continue to do the job that I was currently doing." I had actually changed my hours two years prior so that it would not affect my office practice. The times I was working on the website were the times when I was no longer at the office. I tried to plan everything to allow me to still continue to practice OBGyn at the place I had been working for 16 years and to continue to do surgeries and deliver babies and then on the side to be able to still reach out to women from around the country and give them their treatment on these types of treatment options.

Well, on the Wednesday before Memorial Day, I was practicing at the office and I was told that the leadership wanted me to stay and at 5:00 they were going to meet with me. I called my attorney and he had said he didn't know about the meeting and he had no information and he tried to contact the hospital attorney but was unable to contact the attorney.

At 5:00 PM after all my patients left a team of the leadership from my former employer showed up at the hospital and they said, "Dr. Cly, we appreciate you. We value you. We like you and you've been a very active member of our team for many years." I agreed and said thank you and I felt the same about them as well. But, they said that if I don't turn the website off in 48 hours, then I would be out of a job, and I would be terminated without cause, and I needed to pack my stuff and get out. And if I didn't pack it up 48 hours, then they would have someone pack up my office and all my belongings and ship them to me.

Well, this was a massive shock and totally unexpected. That facts are that on Wednesday before Memorial Day at 5:00, I was told that if I don't turn the website off in 48 hours, by Friday at 5:00PM I would no longer have a job, and I'd be terminated without cause. Also, for the next 90 days I am not allowed to say anything negative about the hospital and that I should recommend all my patients stay at my former employer. I was told that I can't talk about what happened for 90 days. My attorney instructed me to wait 90 days before telling this 'factual narrative' or I could be sued and taken to court. Well, in that meeting, I told the leadership team that I don't want to go down this road, and I hope this doesn't happen and that I still feel like there should be a way where we could work together.

I also let them know that the website and the message of honesty and in speaking the truth and Honest OBGyn information and treatment options is something that I believe in, and that I don't think I'll be turning it off, but I hope that they will reconsider and that we can find a way forward.

So I talked to my attorney and he was trying to work in the background during that 48 hours to see if we could figure out a way to move forward where I could still continue to practice that the same place I had been practicing for 16 years. 48 hours later, was Friday and I had already been asked to help one of my partners with a complex DaVinci surgery because I trained most of my partners and I help them with complex cases. I do the complex prolapse cases that only one other of my 10 partners did, and I trained him as well. So I was doing a DaVinci prolapse case on Friday afternoon approaching the 48 hour deadline. The surgery took about 4 hours, and the case actually didn't finish until 5:30 PM on that Memorial Day Friday.

So after I finished the DaVinci case, I went out to talk with the patient's family, and when I was done talking with the family, I tried to come back in through the surgery area to do my postop orders and my postoperative note and found that my badge didn't work.

They had turned off my access at 5:00 PM, and my badge didn't work. I had to knock on doors and ask people to let me back in to the recovery area so that I could; go to my locker and get my car keys, put in postop orders, and my postop note. Well, when I tried to enter my postop orders and my postdoc note in the computer, I was locked out. My access was disabled and everything was shut down and turned off. I could not enter my orders. I was unable to enter my postop note. I wasn't able to access any of my emails or contacts or anything of that nature. Everything was turned off!

After 16 years, they locked me out like a common criminal at 5:00PM while I was still finishing my surgery and caring for a patient. Really? I had been there for 16 years and helped to create that amazing institution as one of the founding members of the large physicians group. But now, I start a small website where I'm trying to spread the same message that I'd spread for 16 years in that town, trying to spread that message outward to other people in the country and they kick me out like a dirty old shoe that is thrown in the trash.

It had come down to 48 hours and they had said that turn it off or you're out of here. And sure enough, they turned it off at 5:00 and turned me off at 5:00 and locked me out of everything, treating me like a common criminal. I immediately went down to my office, which was down at the other hospital, and luckily there was a door that was open and I was able to get my things out of my office and off the wall. Fortunately my family members came to help. I took down my posters that had been up for 16 years. I took out my knick knacks that had been in my office for 16 years, took out my textbooks that had been sitting there for 16 years. It was all gone, it was all over. They said if I didn't get them out then they would have someone just pack it up and send it to me. And it was a shocking, shocking day, and I pretty much was speechless and in disbelief and couldn't believe that here I was trying to follow the rules and follow the contract, and I spent time, energy, and money with the attorneys to do that. But in a matter of 48 hours they said, "You're gone. You're terminated. Get out of here."

And since that day, which it's been about eight months at this exact point, it's almost as if I am a ghost to most of those people. And I can say that it hurts, it hurts really bad. My patients didn't know what was going on. I didn't even know if this would happen and I couldn't believe that it did happen. Most of my partners didn't even know this was happening. This was on Memorial Day weekend. I had patients scheduled the next week. Monday was off is as it's a national holiday. I think I had a C-section on Tuesday scheduled. I had surgery scheduled the following week. I was so busy that I booked surgeries 3 months out and office visits about 8 weeks out. Also, I had no way to contact these patients. I didn't have any of their records. I didn't have any of their phone numbers. They're all through the central computer. They were contacted later by the staff in the office, and the staff in the office weren't even told about all this. It happened so fast.

So I haven't talked about this much because I had a 90-day gag order that said I wasn't allowed to talk about it, and after that I figured I would wait until I wrote the book and I would put it in the book. And the attorney clarified with my former employer that a factual narrative would be stated after the 90 days. And so this is as factual of a narrative as I can give, and it is what it is right now. And the only thing that makes sense to me as to why this happened, it's the only thing that makes sense because otherwise nothing else makes sense to me.

People ask, "Why did they do that? Why did they let you go? What were they scared of? What was their problem?" Honestly, I am not sure, but I have an idea. I do know that the other hospital in town told me they liked the website and they would love for me to come over there and work. But the problem is that the former employer put me under a two-year non compete clause, which means if I practice in town within two years from this termination, then they would sue me and shut my doors with a lawsuit. And so another hospital said, "Sure, we like the website. We like honesty and transparency and we think you do a good job. You've been an upstanding physician for 16 years in this town with a large following."

And so I asked myself, what was the concern? What was the problem? The only thing I can speculate about is that they were concerned with the idea of trying to sell the educational videos or educational material online, that there was a fear that other doctors in other specialties would also see this idea as something that makes sense and might also try to duplicate it, and that would be something that they were against happening. Other than that, I'm not sure exactly why. Other than that, I have no idea what they were afraid of or how they claim I violated my contract. My attorney's say we did not violate the contract, that is why I hired attorneys. Honestly, I am pretty burnt on attorneys in general right now.

At this point the website has been a labor of love. It is still in its infancy. We're still trying to get off the ground. I am finding that people prefer to use their copay. They prefer to use the health insurance money that they've already paid for and that makes total sense. And so it's not something that is or has been lucrative, but it's something that is a principle of mine and a belief of mine to be able to continue to tell people the honest truth and give them honest OBGyn treatment information.

One last thing, and possibly the REAL reason everything happened the way it did. The only thing that makes 100% sense why this happened is that it has to be God's plan for my life and my wife's life and my family's life. Everything happened in such a way that's so crazy and made no sense that it's got to be God's plan. God is a big part of our life, and our spirituality is very important to us. That's why we named our son Christian, because we felt like he was part of our spiritual journey. And so at this point in time, I am just trying to go with the plan as God is allowing it to unfold and to happen. And I have so far found some.

And so at this point I am just trying to listen for God's plan and trying to allow God's plan to unfold. It has been a tough journey, losing contact with patients who I've known for 16 years and the people that I worked with for many, many years, some of them 16 some of them for several years when they joined the hospital. My wife Megan has been absolutely amazing and the support system who really helped lift me and keep me going during these tough months.

After this happened, I was cut off from everything and couldn't say what happened for the first 90 days. I generally am a positive person. I tried to put a positive spin on the internet and we went ahead and launched the website and we launched the social media and I've been learning that whole aspect of the business and it's a different world and it's been tough, many times it's been very tough. And as I mentioned, Megan has been behind me 100% and many times when I was ready to throw in the towel over the first several months, she was the rock keeping me strong.

Megan was the one who said, "Remember why you started this, remember why we did this. We want women to know the truth. We want them to have the real treatment options. We don't want them to have unnecessary surgeries or in a worst case scenario, we don't want them to go through what your mom and your dad went through." That's why we're doing this, it's to help tell the world that the truth about their options and without her support I definitely would have not been able to continue in this journey. My wife Megan is "small but mighty." She loves with her whole heart and soul through quiet wisdom. I am so thankful for her and for God bringing us together. I love her dearly and couldn't have done this without her.

There's been so many amazing people that I've met along the way. I have been learning new things, I spent the first several months researching all kinds of medical topics and reaching out on the internet. And now I am back in practice again at an amazing place with amazing people in a smaller town that has quality, caring people. I am listening for God's plan every day to see what my next step is. It may be to continue right here at this location, in Rochester, Indiana which is fantastic. It seems like God is placing me where He wants me to go and I'm trying available to the things and the people He's put in front of me every day.

Another really cool thing that happened in the first few months during this journey was being at home and working out of my Worldwide HonestOBGyn Headquarters. It is barn that is in the backyard of our 150 year old farm house that we purchased from Megan's Aunt and Uncle couple of years ago. During the first few months my three year old Christian and our one and a half year old Vicky have been able to come over and hang out during the day and I've been able to be home while working on the website stuff. That has been a really neat opportunity that I've never had before.

Being able to be close with the little ones while working and while trying to do some of the social media and the marketing aspects of the website with the kids running around or nearby has been some valuable time that I will never get back and I'm so grateful for it.

And lastly as I am giving you these details, I'm giving you the details as factually and honestly as I can. And I am able to write this book and without all of these events unfolding, I don't think I would've had the opportunity to write this book. So I look in a positive direction for all the amazing things that God has allowed me to do and to see and to be part of along this journey. And although I miss my patients of 16 years, I have been able to reach out over the internet and discuss educational things and medical OB/GYN topics that I am familiar with and still try to teach and educate women. And I know, although they can't contact me directly because of the non compete clause, and that my former employer owns all of their medical data, and that my former employer has stated

I am never allowed to contact them or ever work with any employee or former employee that I ever worked with, I comforted by the fact that I can still use social media to send my OBGyn knowledge out to the world and somehow that helps me feel connected to them because for 16 years they were like family in many ways and I greatly miss my former patients.

So I don't know what the future holds, but I wish all my former patients well and I thank them all for allowing me to be part of their lives over the years and to care for them and their children and their family. I look forward to what is coming next and I am going to continue being myself and trying to stand up for what's right and trying to keep spreading the message about honest OBGyn treatments.

So when I tell people this story, many of them ask me if I'm going to take legal action or if I'm going to try to fight back and my response to them is the same: "I'm going to tell you; that life is short and I don't think that part of the plan for me is supposed to go into a legal battle. I don't know how much time I have left on this earth and to me it's difficult to go into this type of a fight mode or legal lawsuit mode. And so I'm hopeful that I can continue to do amazing things for people and to try to help people and to stay positive. I guess at this point in time, I feel like God's plan for me is just to continue to keep moving forward. Because going backwards and trying to get into some type of big legal skirmish just doesn't resonate with me as something that I want to do."

Now that being said, if I need to defend myself, then I will do that with every ounce of determination necessary. I am usually someone who will stand up strong and defend a principle and I will do that in as big of a way as I need to versus someone who will start some type of a fight or some type of argument.

That's just the way I've always been. I will certainly defend my patients, I will defend principles, I will defend people who are being taken advantage of and a lot of that goes with how I was raised. So I don't think that a legal battle is something that I want to do or something that I am supposed to do, but I am certainly ready to defend myself if I need to. And at this point in time, there's not much left that my former employer has not stripped from me other than my family and my principles.

This whole project has been really tough and taken a lot of resources. Resources come and go, but family and honesty and principles are something that I value far more than earthly resources.

For My Fellow OB/Gyn Physicians:

I guess one other thing that I want to clarify, even though it's a little bit different or separate from this chapter, it still is something that I want other physicians who might be reading this chapter to know. And that is: if you're a doctor who does not have a DaVinci in your area, then I urge you to offer the women you take care of other minimally invasive procedures and other alternatives than open old-fashioned painful abdominal surgery. And so the goal isn't to try to get everybody to become a DaVinci doctor, the goal is to allow women to have all their treatment options. And for those doctors out there who are still doing outdated old fashioned abdominal hysterectomies without really offering a vaginal approach or really offering a laparoscopic surgery to your patients, then please consider what you're doing and would you do the same for your mother or would you do the same for your wife?

I think it's important that we all continue as doctors to learn and to do new things. We know things change. We have to learn new things for our board exams every year. So if you're a doctor who's out there and you think I'm only trying to tell everyone you have to do DaVinci, that is not my goal. But I do want to encourage you to offer your patients the latest up to date treatments that's in their best interest.

And lastly, my hope for my fellow OB/GYN's is that as we move forward and as HonestOBGyn.com moves forward; I hope we can come together as OB/GYNs who are practicing honesty and help develop a camaraderie and collegiality of other OB/GYNs who are trying to do the best for their patients and who can help each other learn new skills to make sure that we're doing the best for our patients. The more we can help each other, the more we can help our patients. I think that is really the most important message I want to tell my fellow OB/GYNs.

For Women Everywhere:

The video that I created, found on my homepage, focuses on the DaVinci, because that's the beginning of this journey for me. When you go to my homepage, HonestOBGyn.com, you'll see a professional video that I created and it goes through some of 'my why'. I don't want anyone to suffer like my family and I suffered at the hands of bad doctors. And, I want patients to know how to recognize 'red flags" by empowering them with information. I know there still are the doctors who try to tell the patients that they're not candidates and they're going to try "bait & switch" or mislead, like the doctors I mentioned. This is another reason why HonestOBGyn.com has a physician directory for you to be able to put in your zip code and find doctors who are doing up to date treatments with DaVinci's anywhere in the country. I know that there are doctors who are in other areas of the country who will try to tell you, you can't have that done. As a doctor, I know you can have it done almost everywhere, you just got to know where to look. I want you to know where to look and am giving you that information.

After 20+ years in this profession, I have worked to improve the quality of women's health care by focusing on teaching and guiding doctors. I now realize that in addition to helping doctors, the patients have to have transparency, specific information, and step by step treatment options in order to bring transparency to this specialty. For one reason: doctors cannot hide behind privacy laws or misinformation - the transparency will drive honesty and the truth. The other things to revolutionize surgical transparency is what HonestOBGyn.com has in the works and it will be coming out soon. I'm very excited about these things. These future modules will help to change the perception of physicians as well as enhance the trust that patients have in us doctors. What HonestOBGyn.com has planned is going to give you information that up until now, has never been published. This information has never been available to the public, anywhere in the world. For the first time you will know the real truth about the doctors you choose, how good they really are. You will be guaranteed truth and transparency, before you ever make an appointment or choose your doctor.

5 Decrease the Cost of Care, but Let a Few Teenagers Die

One of the things that has been occurring over the course of my career, that I noticed when I was a resident back in 1996 to 2000, is the shift from taking caring for the individual woman versus controlling the care and cost of care for all women. In this section I'm going to talk about the underlying current that's been occurring over the past 20 years. That is, the money is driving the healthcare industry and dictating the treatment goals which is now an accepted thought process. Additionally, it has affected the physicians and what treatment we choose, because we have to include a financial consideration to the type of treatment provided to a patient. My hope with this section is that you will become aware of the constraints that the overall system is placing on your care and know if it is affecting your ability to heal and get back to the life that you love. In addition, some ways to ensure you get the best care possible (not just the cheapest) because the individual patient and their treatment is really what should be the overriding factor. Let me explain that a little bit because that to me sounds confusing as I am writing it here. So this is one example of finances controlling the care: pap smears.

A pap smear is a test that's done at the time of an annual examination for women. It's a swab of the cervix inside the vagina, checking for any precancerous cells that could lead to cervical cancer. There've been a lot of changes in the last 20 years on the guidelines of pap smears, the frequency of pap smears, how they're done. And what is the goal of pap smears? As many of you may remember, it was always thought that a pap smear had to be done every single year. Many women still want to have their pap smear done every year. Women come in for the annual exam, which I still think is a good idea and is still recommended. This includes the breast exam, a full body exam history, a pelvic exam, and a discussion of overall health. So many women think the annual exam is just a pap smear, but a pap smear is just one of the many parts of an annual exam. Studies have been done in the past 10 - 15 years looking at the cost of doing pap smears on everyone in America every year compared to the cost of the cancers and the detection rate of cancers of the cervix. And then comparing that to the frequency of the pap smear detecting cancers and how successful an annual pap smear is on everyone. These studies showed that the cost of doing pap smears on every single woman every year, far exceeds the cost of doing pap smears every couple, three, or five years. Versus the cost of some women developing cancer and having cancer treatments if pap smears are not done every year. Looking at those side by side, studies showed that there's a lot of money spent on yearly pap smears and associated procedures from those. And by spreading the pap smear to every several years, there would be a lot of money saved and <u>not many cancers missed</u>. Nice, right?...

Now, you notice I said <u>not many cancers missed</u> by following the less frequent guidelines. "They" (the committee that recommends and pushes these new medical pap smear guidelines) tell us doctors that adopting this new, less frequent pap smear policy the medical systeom is going to save a significant amount of money, cut down on a significant number of followup procedures, and not dramatically increase the cancer rate. However, the tradeoff is that there will be some people whose cancer will be missed and these people will develop cancer with this new every three - five year pap smear guideline. BUT, the cost of the cancer care for those people and the treatment of the missed cancers is much less costly overall than the total cost to the medical system overall if we'd still continue to do pap smears every year.

That is a major example and a major frustration for me because I became a doctor to help people heal. I became a doctor and took an oath to do no harm and to help women. My concern is the women that I take care of in my office, the women that see me as their doctor. And my concern is making sure that they don't get cancer in their cervix. And so that puts my ethics at odds with the rules the system is trying to enforce because it is very important to me to make sure that the patients I take care of and who trust me with their healthcare and trust me to help them avoid cancer, do not get cancer because of the new guidelines that are being pushed upon OB-GYNs in America. And ultimately, if I followed those guidelines, then there's a chance some of my patients who place their trust in me will end up having cancer. So, in order to be a "good doctor" and bridge that ethics gap, I individualize the patients needs, history, goals, and family history with the guidelines and come up with a personalized plan for each patient instead of a blanket generic policy. The American College of Obstetrics and Gynecology states that for all the 15-19 year old teenage girls, ONLY 1-2 of them out of 1,000,000 will get cervical cancer so therefore we don't need to start pap smears until they are 21 years old.......Hold up.....only 1-2 of them....

Needless to say, this is unacceptable to me. It's not something that I could ever live with and not something that in my heart, or my belief in honesty and transparency that I can not tell you the truth about. I don't want any of my patients to get cervical cancer. I'm trying to help my patients heal or prevent problems and take care of them the way I would want to be taken care of. And so that's an example of a massive shift that's occurred in medicine. And so you might be wondering, why did this happen? What it sounds crazy and here's, here's part of the explanation.

One of the problems with the abnormal pap smear situation is that there are several ways to do a pap smear and there's several companies that have lab testing procedures and machines to check for pap smears and there's profit in all of these things. And so you've got several companies trying to come up with the best pap smear test. But there is more than one way to do pap smears. Additionally, when a pap smear shows there was an abnormal finding, then the next step usually is a procedure called a colposcopy. And we have you come back into the office, we do a pelvic exam and use a tool that looks like a microscope and we can zoom in on the cervix and look at it. Also, we put some vinegar solution on the cervix. And if there's abnormal changes to the cells in the skin on your cervix, then that could indicate some precancerous areas specifically. And we then might take biopsies or do a procedure to remove abnormal cells. The colposcopy really zooms in on the exact area to find where that abnormal pap smear result came from because the original pap smear doesn't say your entire cervix is abnormal. It just highlights that somewhere on your cervix there are some microscopic cells that might be abnormal.

So, okay, that sounds reasonable, right?.....It does to me. But the cost of the colposcopy is much higher than a pap smear. So a colposcopy generally is $300-$500 hundred dollars. Any biopsies we do an additional hundreds of dollars, so a colposcopy could end up costing in the thousands. Part of the reason financially why the guidelines are changing because what the system is saying is that too many people are getting Colposcopic examinations and charges and that turn out to be negative and that's unnecessary. And they're also saying that as a result of this, too many people were also then being subjected to surgical procedures of the cervix that are likely unnecessary given the new understanding of cervical cancer and HPV in pap smear results and all the new in technology information we have. So, on the one hand, that does make sense. I certainly don't want anyone to go through unnecessary surgeries or unnecessary procedures, but on the other hand, applying a blanket statement to all women that you don't need a pap smear, except for every three years based on your age is also questionable to me.

Last thing on this, not to get too deep into it, which I may already have, because this is a soapbox of mine. It seems like every six to seven years, a new committee is formed about pap smears. And it comes out and says, okay, doctors, the committee just met and made a decision. 'We, the smart committee people in our profession have decided that we are no longer gonna do pap smear screening the way we did for the last seven years. It's all changing. We're going to do it this way now because this way is better. And the way we did it for the past 6 to 7 years was not good.' I say this because I've been in the game since 1996 as a resident. I started med school in 1992. So I've seen this happen a couple times and I'm just frustrated.

I guess as a doctor who has been doing this a long time and it just is frustrating telling someone the party line and then a few years later having to say, "I'm sorry I was totally wrong. They've changed everything and everything I told you for the last six, seven, eight years, just disregard it." And maybe that's because I have patients that have been with me for for 16 or even 20 years. I've been in my last location for 16 years and I have a couple of patients who come to me from Ohio and I've known them for 20 years. It is frustrating as a doctor to tell them what you believe in your heart and they trust you and then come back and tell them later, I'm sorry I was told to tell you something else now. Also, everything I told you before was wrong. I know that may be just the way it is and we are always learning new things in the system. But it's frustrating to me as a doctor and someone who patients trust. I try to tell my patients, I tried to do the best I can do and I want the best for them. Maybe I'm placing too much hope in the system. Maybe I'm placing too much thought into this, but that's who I am and I care about my patients. I stress about them. I worry about them at night, and about their babies and I want the best for them. It's because I care, but that's who I am and that's just the way it is and I'm not complaining about that. Actually caring is what helps me do the best job I can for my patients.

Another example of the cost being more important than patients or in this case a baby. In this next example, it involves accepting and allowing a baby to die. This was the first time I realized in my professional career that financially driven treatment guidelines and recommendations were occurring. This was way back when I was a resident between the years of 1996 and 2000. At the time I read this study and report I felt like I had been brainwashed and I was trying to wake up from this craziness. Just like as if I was in a movie called the matrix. And I had just taken a little capsule, like the lead star in that movie, and woke up from a self-imposed virtual reality world where the robots had taken over.

When I saw this next example and study, I'm going to tell you, I was mortified, horrified, and I thought: "Oh my gosh, is this what is being taught to us? And how much of this garbage am I believing?" And it made me open my eyes and question things - so that when I'm told new things or taught new things, I have to think internally, okay, is this really in the best interest of the patient? And if it is not, what parts of it are, ethically, acceptable and what parts need to be challenged so that I may continue to perform as a physician ethically and uphold the Hippocratic oath to my patients.

I remember being in labor and delivery reading this article and it was an article comparing the costs of vaginal birth after cesarean sections compared to flat out repeat cesarean sections. And so what does that mean? That means that if a woman has a cesarean section for whatever reason, the next time she has a baby, trying to allow her to have a vaginal birth again after a cesarean section in the last pregnancy. And that's called a VBAC. The article in the research study looked at the following: What happens when comparing repeat VBACs for everyone vs repeat Cesarean Sections for everyone? They added up how much did the repeat C-sections cost, how much did their postpartum postoperative care costs if there were any challenges with the babies, or injuries, what were those total costs? And then they compared that to the cost of a same number of women who attempted a vaginal birth after cesarean section. Many of those were successful and they had a vaginal delivery. Some of those were not successful. They ended up having to have a C-section and some of those ruptured their uterus during labor because there is a risk of the incision rupturing during a VBAC of about 1.5% And they looked at those women who had a uterine rupture during labor, how much were the costs to fix that. And in those cases where a uterine rupture occurs, it can be a disastrous outcome for the baby and frequently includes death or mental handicap for the baby if it lives. They looked at those costs as well and for the long term care for those infants. And then they took the cost of malpractice lawsuits for the babies that died. Then they added all of this up together and came up with a recommendation. What this study showed was that it is cheaper to let women attempt a VBAC and pay for the lawsuit costs of the dead babies that occurred during the VBACs and it was more expensive to just do repeat Cesarean sections. It didn't matter that babies don't die during a repeat Cesarean section. So after this recommendation was to allow women to have VBACs because it's going to be cheaper overall. Even if some of their babies die, it still saves a lot of money for the system.

Wow! When I read that, I was mortified. I thought this was ridiculous. Who is callous enough to think about this and then try to do a study and come up with a plan to save money for the system. But in doing so, allow babies to die and just say, well, it's okay because we have saved money overall. That was shocking to me and that's when I felt like I woke up from a weird dream. I said to myself, I'm not going to continue to be brainwashed the rest of my life. And so that has dictated a lot of how I look at things because I don't want my patients to be the ones to have their baby go through a horrible situation or outcome or develop cancer from a pap smear guideline that allows some women to develop cancer. I went into medicine to help people. I didn't go into medicine to save money for the insurance company or someone else just so a CEO can get a bigger bonus at the end of the year.

Now that being said, I'm definitely trying to be considerate of how much money I spend and that's very important. And so I want everyone to know that it is not appropriate to spend as much money as you can and get as many treatments as you can. But it is appropriate to individualize a persons a care plan and their situation and order tests or labs or come up with treatments that will serve them the best in light of their, their personal situation to help them heal and get back to living the life that they love. And along with that, it's always important to docent these things as well.

Now, some doctors might read this and claim that I am trying to say that all other doctors other than me are callous and greedy and trying to milk the system. If you are a physician and you're reading this right now and you're thinking that, well then you're interpreting my words in your own way. Either because I'm not conveying my point well enough, or you may have some internal turmoil over the words I'm saying in the financial considerations in medicine that you have experienced. So for you, the women reading this, I want you to know that I'm not trying to paint other doctors as bad people who are trying to just make a lot of money. Actually, most doctors are not like that. Most doctors care about their patients. Most doctors are overwhelmed and trying to catch up to the busy-ness of the ever-changing guidelines and system and the computers as well as take care of their own families at home. It's a rat race. And so these words I'm saying are so that you as patients will know how to understand the behind the scenes stuff. And for the doctors who are listening or reading this, I want you to understand where I'm coming from and I hope you will be able to feel empowered by knowing there are other doctors out there who are frustrated like you are. Because I sure am.

Those doctors who feel like me, I suspect we got into this because of our desire to help people. Unfortunately the system is continually trying to change things up. Now, are there bad doctors out there? Yes there are. Are there greedy doctors out there? Yes there are. I know several of them, but they are the minority of doctors.

Now, on the other hand, if you're reading this and you are a doctor who approves of five o'clock friday C-sections, or you're a doctor who baits and switches patients to higher profit treatments, or you're a doctor who just doesn't care and you are in this for the money, or if your doctor is burned out and because of burnout, you no longer have compassion for your patients; -----> I urge you to look inside yourself and look at your situation and figure out how you can change your behaviors rise up to the level of the Hippocratic oath, rise up to the level that you come from a place of truth and transparency and can make a difference for patients and put them first.

I know that there are some people in every profession that are not going to change. There are some people who just care about the money. There are people who are gonna read this and angrily disagree and then throw this book away or throw it in the fire because they don't like what I'm saying. Either way, I know that I am stating the truth and speaking from my heart, I'm speaking it from the experience that I've seen since starting med school in 1992 and practicing as an OBGyn for the last 20+ years.

6 What is the BIG idea?
How This Book WILL Improve Your Life

The big idea for this book is that the information in this book is a valuable resource that you will be able to go to when you or a loved one faces an OBGyn problem. And you want or need the most up to date vital information to allow you to get the best treatment, avoid unnecessary surgeries and heal in the best way possible to get back to the life that you love. And even years after this book is published, I want you to know that you can always go to HonestOBGyn.com for information that is truthful and up to date about every OBGyn topic. I want to help guide you through the knowledge. Why is it so important? This information is so important because it will continue to change over time with new, better treatments and there will be updates which will be available on HonestOBGyn.com Doctors are always learning and there will always be some doctors who are not keeping up with the current knowledge. And there will be some doctors who may not have the resources available to perform certain treatments. So it is even more important that you know what all the treatment options are and be able to ask about these other treatments. Also, if it's reasonable or necessary, for you to travel to some place where the treatments are available. I think that brings up a good point in that I'm not trying to recommend every patient has to have the newest, fanciest treatment because, there are ways to treat someone in a very effective way without the latest and greatest treatment. But there are also times where the latest treatment is necessary and traveling a couple of hours can make all the difference in the world.

For example, the DaVinci robotic surgery system s is a good example of what I'm trying to explain. There are many surgeries that can be done with the DaVinci system that could also be done by someone who does advanced laparoscopic surgeries. So there is overlap, and you could get the same minimally invasive procedure with a doctor who performs advanced laparoscopy and not need the Da Vinci system. But, you have to know this information and that is exactly what HonestOBGyn.com and I am trying to do.

Most doctors don't do regular advanced laparoscopy anymore because many doctors have the availability of the DaVinci technology. Remember, some doctors in places without the DaVinci will lean toward an open procedure because it's easier, they do it more often, it's faster, and oh ...yeah ... and it also pays better.

Therefore, in those places an open abdominal procedure might be the standard of care for that town. These are the cases where the HonestOBGyn.com knowledge is extremely important for you and will help you find a minimally invasive surgeon or surgery. HonestOBGyn.com is building the database of surgeons who do these types of procedures so that you'll be able to find that information easily and search by zip code to be able to see what are the abilities of the doctors in your area.

7 Hysterectomy, Sometimes Unnecessary & Sometimes a Lifesaver!

Hysterectomy, sometimes unnecessary and sometimes a lifesaver. So the big idea with the information in this chapter is I want you to have all of the knowledge about hysterectomy and other procedures that let you avoid it as well as the reasons and evaluation all in one place, in a complete package.

I want it to be similar to as if you are talking to me in an educational seminar and told me the diagnosis you were given and then I would tell you what most up to date treatment options are for that problem. The ins and outs so you can know if your doctor is guiding you to the treatment that is best for you. What's new and different with HonestOBGyn.com and Dr. Geoffrey Cly's Pocket Guides, is that I created these for hysterectomy and other OBGyn problems as well as personal video seminars that follow along. And it is me explaining to you personally, the details about hysterectomies as well as avoiding them that I'm going to tell you in this chapter. I want you to get back to living the life that you love.

My hope is that with this knowledge, you will be empowered with information and you'll feel reassured, less anxiety, less frustration, and know the best path to get heal from the problems you're having.

I want you to feel similar to my patients and how they feel many times when they leave my office after a visit. Many of my patients have told me over the past 20 years, "Dr. Cly, just talking to you and having you tell me my options has made me feel so much better, taken away my nervousness, my anxiety, my frustration and giving me hope that I can feel good again." That's what I've heard from my patients. And that's what I want you to have after reading this chapter.

So one example about avoiding an unnecessary hysterectomy I'll share with you is from a close personal friend of mine. I have taken care of his wife for many years and delivered their children. Several years ago she started having challenges of bleeding and cramping. So my buddy called me and said, "Hey, can you take a look at my wife? She's really struggling. This stuff is really affecting her ability to take care of the family. She can't get out of bed sometimes and she just doesn't know what to do." So of course I said sure, "I can evaluate her and what's going on."

Side note: I take care of my friend's wives? Really.....well yes, but it's very likely that my "friends" only want to be my friend because they want me to give free medical care to their wives and save money by asking me questions at any time, day or night. Oh well, ... this is my reality and I do take care of many, many of my friends wives. Heck, maybe it is the only way I can keep friends? Who knows for sure, lol. (Can I put lol in a book?) Anyways, I think it's because they trust me and gotten to know me over the years and feel confident I will care for their wives like I would want to be cared for. Who knows?

Either way, when I asked her to come into the office to see me, she wanted a hysterectomy. She was just tired of the bleeding and cramping and she couldn't live her life. She was in bed all weekend when the symptoms happened. She was missing activities with her kids. She was unable to take care of them during the day. And it affected them both as far as the intimacy in there relationship. They were unable to have sex or be intimate very often because of the bleeding and cramping. And so like most women come in to see me with these challenges, she wanted a hysterectomy.

Now she was a younger woman in the sense of she was in her thirties and other than the bleeding and cramping, she hadn't tried many things yet. This is common for many women because you are busy with life and taking care of others and your family. Many women, possibly like you tolerate a lot of symptoms for a long time before getting very frustrated. By the time she came in to see me, she was "over it" and just want her uterus taken out. So what I did with her is what I'm going to share with you. In this next part of the chapter I will walk through these different possibilities and options. In her case, we ended up determining that for her symptoms, her goals, her activities, and her busy life; the best thing for her would be an endometrial ablation.

Before I go into the details for you about an ablation and other options, I should let you know how things turned out. She had that procedure several years ago. She got her life back. Her bleeding is gone and the cramping is minimal. She still has her uterus and she is living the life that she wanted to live. She was able to keep her uterus and avoid a hysterectomy. I want you to know that that information for when you go to see your doctor.

When you go to your doctor, please feel free to show him or her The HonestOBGyn.com, Dr.

Geoffrey Cly's Pocket Guide for Hysterectomy. I encourage you to say, "Here's the options I saw from this website called HonestOBGyn.com. I'm interested in these options and I think I really want to talk about....." I know that with this information, you may be able to avoid a hysterectomy, or get the correct hysterectomy and get back to the life that you love.

I want you to have Dr. Geoffrey Cly's Pocket Guide for Hysterectomy. I listed it below and I encourage you to consider going to HonestOBGyn.com to sign up for access to the personalized video where I walk you through the symptoms, answer questions, and you are guided to the best treatments. In addition to that, many women have found the private HonestOBGyn Members Facebook group extremely valuable. In that private group I am giving live educational seminars and answering questions directly for members 24/7. It is kind of like having a 'Doctor in your pocket'.

First off, here are my important thoughts regarding hysterectomy:

Dr. Cly's important recommendations
- No matter what path it should be personalized for you.
- Younger patients should avoid a hysterectomy with these exceptions,
  - You are finished having children.
  - You "just can't take this anymore"
- Many OBGyn have DaVinci laparoscopic experience.
- Choose an OBGyn who perform DaVinci surgeries or Laparoscopic surgeries or Vaginal surgeries if you're considering a hysterectomy.

- Be wary of an OBGyn recommending a painful large incision, otherwise known as an abdominal hysterectomy.
- You usually don't need a large incision and we OBGyns get paid more money to do surgery with a large incision.

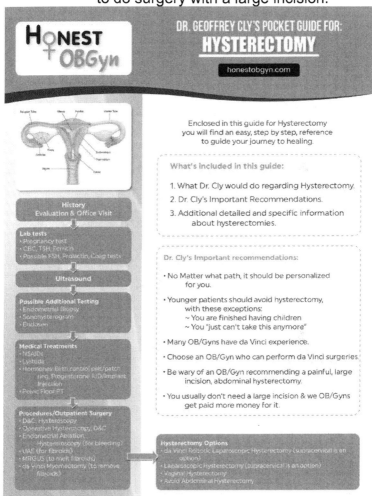

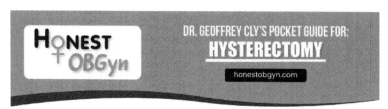

If you have been recommended to have a Hysterectomy, then the following information will help guide you on your journey to becoming healthy again. This fact sheet focuses on standard of care, treatment options in the United States. Even though not every treatment may be ideal for your situation, your doctor or provider should educate you about all of them, so you can make an informed decision.

The following information is listed in chronological steps that should happen from the first visit. These steps should be followed prior to performing a hysterectomy. Some of these steps will apply to you and some may not apply. There are different Gyn problems that can be resolved with a Hysterectomy. If you want more info on the other problems, please go to HonestOBGyn.com.

1. **Detailed History and Examination**
2. **Blood Tests:**
    a. Almost always ordered: Pregnancy test, Complete Blood Count (CBC), Thyroid Stimulating Hormone (TSH), Ferritin.
    b. Ordered based on other symptoms: Follicle Stimulating Hormone (FSH), Prolactin, Coagulation testing.
3. **Imaging:** Ultrasound (most common), but also possible are MRI, or CT
4. **Additional Possible Testing:**
    a. Endometrial Biopsy usually when > 35 years old and having break through bleeding.
    b. **Sonohysterogram:** This is an ultrasound with saline to evaluate endometrial lining for polyps/fibroids.
    c. **Endosee:** A very small camera that can be inserted in through cervix in the office to directly look at the interior uterine lining, called the endometrium.
5. **Important Factors before moving on:**
    a. If there is cancer, then consult a Gynecologic Oncologist.
    b. If your symptoms stem from Abnormal Uterine Bleeding, Endometriosis, Fibroids, Pelvic Prolapse, or Ovarian Cysts, then refer to the HonestOBGyn.com and select one of those Pocket Guides or Treatment Options and Pathways for specific information about each of those problems.
6. **Medical Treatments:** That may help prevent or postpone a hysterectomy:
    a. **Non-hormonal medications:**
        i. NSAIDs (Ibuprofen, Naproxen, etc..) to lighten amount of menstrual bleeding, and decrease cramps.

ii. Lysteda: Tranexamenic acid tablets taken 3x per day during your menses to dramatically decrease amount of bleeding

b. **Hormonal medications:** will decrease menstrual bleeding and decrease cramps

i. Birth control hormones: (Pills, Patches, Vaginal Ring) may be used even if tubes are tied in some cases

ii. Progesterone only: (Depo-Provera, Nexplanon, Intra-Uterine Devices) also may be considered if tubes are tied.

c. **Pelvic Floor Physical Therapy:** (for pelvic prolapse or pelvic pain) Physical therapy with a specific Women's Pelvic Floor Trained Therapist may help decrease prolapse and improve pelvic pain.

7. **Same Day Outpatient Procedures & Outpatient Surgery Options:** These may be able to correct the problem in order to avoid a hysterectomy.

a. **D&C, Hysteroscopy:** this stabilizes and stops the current bleeding, but does not help prevent any future bleeding.

b. **Operative Hysteroscopy** - shaves down any fibroids protruding through middle lining of uterus and removes thick menstrual lining. Pregnancy is still possible in the future.

c. **Endometrial Ablation, Hysteroscopy:** (for abnormal uterine bleeding) Permanently removes and seals menstrual lining to prevent future periods. It is not safe to become pregnant after this procedure.

i. Excellent option, works very well, minimal recovery time, same day procedure.

ii. If less than 40 years old, then it may only last several years before bleeding starts again.

iii. Higher chance of a future hysterectomy if <40 years old, but it is minimally invasive, minimal recovery, 1-3 days off work, a good 1st step to consider.

iv. Ablation not recommended after menopause, usually around 52 years old.

d. **Uterine Artery Embolization** – (for fibroids) fibroid arteries blocked, they dissolve, future pregnancy possible.

e. **MRI guided ultrasound** – (for fibroids) newer procedure, MRI "melts" fibroids, only in select cities, may not be covered under insurance, but may be an excellent option to consider. Future pregnancy possible.

f. **Myomectomy** – (for fibroids) easily done with da Vinci Robotic Laparoscopic system in most cases. Allows for future pregnancy. Home same day, driving next day, off work 1-3 weeks. Wait one year before attempting pregnancy. Future pregnancy desire is not required for a myomectomy.

8. **Hysterectomy:**

a. **Considerations:**

- Off work times are 1 week up to 6 weeks.
- Many women go back to work in 1-2 weeks. Many jobs grant 6 weeks off of work for a hysterectomy, no matter what type.
- Abdominal Hysterectomy will require 4-6 weeks off of work and no driving for 2 weeks
- No sex for 6-8 weeks except with Supracervical Hysterectomy

honestobgyn.com

- **Ovaries:**
  - a) Keep your ovaries if they are normal, functioning, and you are pre-menopausal.
  - b) If you are around or in menopause, then ovarian removal is a consideration – discuss with your doctor.
  - c) If your ovaries are a source of recurrent pain, cysts, adhesions, anxiety about future cancer, or you have a family history of ovarian cancer –discuss options with your doctor.
    - i. Sometimes removing 1 ovary and leaving one is a consideration.
- b. **Vaginal Hysterectomy** - entire surgery performed through vagina, less pain. Driving next day.
- c. **da Vinci Robotic Laparoscopic Hysterectomy** - advanced laparoscopic system, precision movements, less bleeding, small incisions, less pain, home same day or next day.
- d. **Laparoscopic Assisted Vaginal Hysterectomy** - laparoscope used to separate uterus, then surgery completed through vagina. Home next day, driving next day.
- e. **Supracervical Hysterectomy** - Uterus removed with laparoscope, da Vinci, or laparotomy (large incision), but the cervix remains at the top of the vagina. More information can be found here:
  www.honestobgyn.com/supracervical-hysterectomy/
  - Your pelvic floor support at the cervix stays intact unlike other hysterectomy types.
  - da Vinci Supracervical Hysterectomy heals faster.
  - No stitches in vagina and sex is possible as soon as you feel like it.
- f. **Abdominal Hysterectomy**
  - Rarely needs to be performed any longer and should not be offered routinely.
  - Easier surgery for physician, much harder for you.
  - Doctor gets paid more money even though this is like "Your Grandmother's hysterectomy".
  - Large, painful incision, a 3 day stay in hospital, 6-week recovery, and no driving for 2 weeks.
  - Unfortunately, outdated doctors are still routinely recommending it.

References
ACOG Committee on Practice Bulletins. (2008, August). Alternatives to Hysterectomy in the Management of Leiomyomas. Retrieved from American Congress of Obstetricians and Gynecologists: www.acog.org
ACOG Committee on Practice Bulletins. (2013, July). Management of Abnormal Uterine Bleeding Associated with Ovulatory Dysfunction. Retrieved from American College of Obstetricians and Gynecologists: http://www.acog.org
Andrew M. Kaunitz, M. (2017, November 28). Approach to abnormal uterine bleeding in nonpregnant reproductive-age women. Retrieved from UpToDate: http://www.uptodate.com
Committee on Gynecologic Practice. (2013, April). Management of Acute Abnormal Uterine Bleeding in Nonpregnant Reproductive-Aged Women. Retrieved from American College of Obstetricians and Gynecologists: http://www.acog.org
Committee on Gynecologic Practice. (2017, June). Committee Opinion: Choosing the Route of Hysterectomy for Benign Disease. Retrieved from American College of Obstetricians and Gynecologists: acog.org
Committee on Practice Bulletins -Gynecology and American Urogynecologic Societys, Tulikangas, MD, Paul. (2017, November). ACOG Practice Bulletin Pelvic Organ Prolapse, Number 185. Retrieved from The American College of Obstetricians and Gynecologists: www.acog.org
Elizabeth A. Stewart, M. (2017, June 5). Overview of treatment of uterine leiomyomas (fibroids). Retrieved from Uptodate.com: http://uptodate.com
Geoffrey C. Cly, M. (2018, 1 28). Expert Opinion and Current Practice Standards. Fort Wayne, Indiana.

honestobgyn.com

This Pocket Guide is one of many examples I have created for multiple different types of OBGyn problems. The other ones are available at HonestOBGyn.com and discuss things like Endometriosis, Pelvic Pain, Ovarian Cysts, Pelvic Prolapse, Heavy Bleeding, Uterine Fibroids, Preventing Miscarriages, Protecting Your Unborn Baby until Delivery, and more.

8 Fireballs, Fibroids, and an Amazing Woman's Journey

I want to tell you about one of my early patients who had a significant amount of uterine fibroids. This was back in 2007. I had a lady come to me and she had heard about me using the robotic surgery system. And at that time I had not done a complex DaVinci Robotic Myomectomy, (removal of fibroids and fixing the uterus back to normal) on a uterus with a large amount of fibroids. A woman came to see me and she had about 20 fibroids. Her uterus was absolutely riddled with fibroids and it was the most fibroids I think I had ever seen as a younger doctor. And I simply told her, "Look, I don't want you to be my guinea pig. Because I have only done a couple robotic myomectomies." Also that is why she came to me, she wanted a robotic myomectomy. I said, "I don't think I'm good enough to do this surgery like you want. And I don't know if anybody can do it Robotically with that many fibroids." I just didn't know if it could be done. She appreciated my honesty and she asked if I knew anyone who might try to do it Robotically with the DaVinci system. I said, "Ya know, I do know one guy, and he is the best in the world. He is only a couple of hours away from here. I am happy to check with him and ask him about this case and give you his number."

So I called a colleague who helped train me on the DaVinci. This person was Arnold Advincula, MD. Dr. Arnold Advincula Advincula is one of the first robotic experts in the world. He trained most of us "early adopters" on the DaVinci in person, on videos, and at live DaVinci surgical conferences. Dr. Arnold Advincula was at the University of Michigan at that time. And I called him and I said, "Hey, Arnie, here's what I got. I don't even know if it's possible, but what do you think?" He said, "I think it's possible, we've done a lot of myomectomies." At the time he was number one in the world for DaVinci robotic surgery for gynecology. He was teaching all of us DaVinci Gynecologists in America. This guy is an amazing physician, a wonderful person, and very humble. I will always be thankful for his mentoring and teaching.

So back to the story. I gave her his number and she made an appointment with Dr. Advincula. What happened next absolutely blew my mind!! This patient scheduled a DaVinci Laparoscopic Myomectomy with Dr. Advincula. However, not only did he remove more than 20 fibroids, but he sent her home the same day! And she did great! It was absolutely amazing. This is back in 2007, back in the early days of DaVinci when people were just beginning to unleash the power of the DaVinci Surgical System. I was flabbergasted. She hardly had any pain. She was able to save her uterus and in 2008 after waiting the recommended year to heal, she got pregnant. I delivered her first baby in 2008 and her second child in 2014. I still know her to this day, she is an amazing woman. What is so incredible is that the DaVinci allowed her to get a minimally invasive procedure, go home the same day, and then become a mother of 2 amazing children without having a hysterectomy or a lot of pain and suffering with the myomectomy.

So a DaVinci Myomectomy, as you can see from her amazing example is something that works very well. Additionally, most people only have a few fibroids. One of the challenges with fibroids is that they will try to come back after several years in many people. We don't completely understand why they occur, but if you have several fibroids, most likely you're going to get some other fibroids in other areas in your uterus in the future. Sometimes they stabilize and they don't cause problems, but sometimes they continue to grow. So a myomectomy is a great option if you want to keep your uterus. There are other options that you should know about.

In this next Guide, Dr. Geoffrey Cly's Comprehensive Guide For Uterine Fibroids, I discuss fibroids and the options to remove them, melt them, shrink them, as well as take them and the uterus out with a hysterectomy.

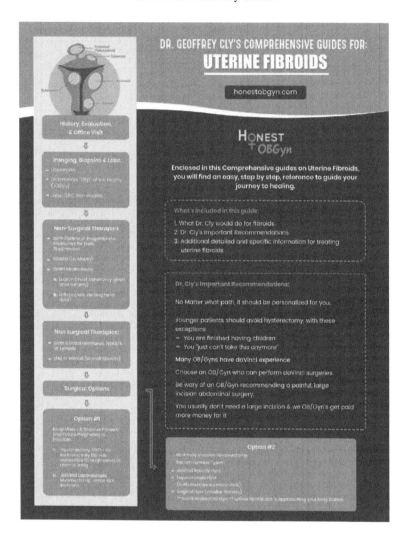

WAIT! Don't Take My Uterus!

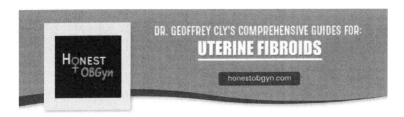

If you have been diagnosed with Uterine Fibroids, then the following information will help guide you on your journey to becoming healthy again. This fact sheet focuses on standard of care, treatment options in the United States. Even though not every treatment may be ideal for your situation, your doctor or provider should educate you about all of them, so you can make an informed decision.

The following information is listed in chronological steps that should happen from the first visit:

1. **Detailed History and Examination**
2. **Imaging:** Ultrasound (most common), but also possible are MRI, or CT, or Endosee intra-uterine camera
3. **In Office Endometrial Biopsy** – only needed in some cases

4. **Medical Treatments & Procedure Options**
   a. Hormonal medications
      - Birth control hormones: (Pills, Patches, Vaginal Ring)
      - Progesterone only: (Depo-Provera, Nexplanon, Intra-Uterine Devices)
   b. Non-hormonal medications
      - NSAIDs (Ibuprofen, Naproxen, etc.) and/or Lysteda
   c. Operative Hysteroscopy – shaves down the fibroids protruding through middle lining of uterus.
      • If done with Ablation – It is not safe to become pregnant after this procedure.
   d. Uterine Artery Embolization – fibroid arteries blocked, they dissolve, future pregnancy possible.
   e. MRI guided ultrasound – newer procedure, MRI "melts" fibroids, only in select cities, may not be covered under insurance, but may be reasonable option.
      Future pregnancy possible.

5. **Surgical Options** – divided in 2 categories
   a. Uterine Sparing (Keep your Uterus)
      - Myomectomy – easily done with daVinci Robotic Laparoscopic system. In past was done with open laparotomy incision. Allows for future pregnancy.
   b. Uterine Removal (Hysterectomy)
      - **Vaginal Hysterectomy** - entire surgery performed through vagina, less pain.
      - **daVinci Robotic Laparoscopic Hysterectomy** – advanced laparoscopic system, precision movements, less bleeding, small incisions, less pain.
      - **Laparoscopic Assisted Vaginal Hysterectomy** – laparoscope used to separate uterus, then surgery completed through vagina.
         • **More information can be found here: www.honestobgyn.com/supracervical-hysterectomy/**
      - Your ovary should be preserved and fixed if possible.

- **Laparoscopy:**
  - Cyst removal and reconstruction of ovary – must have a daVinci robotic laparoscopic system to be able to do this.
  - Cyst wall removal and allow ovary to heal on its own – acceptable for smaller cysts, this is the only option if a daVinci robotic laparoscopic system is not available

- **Abdominal Hysterectomy**
  - Rarely needs to be performed any longer and should not be offered routinely.
  - Easier surgery for physician, much harder for you.
  - Doctor gets paid more money even though this is like "Your Grandmother's hysterectomy".
  - Large, painful incision, a 3 day stay in hospital, 6-week recovery, and no driving for 2 weeks.
  - Unfortunately, outdated doctors are still routinely recommending it.

References:

ACOG Committee on Practice Bulletins. (2008, August). *Alternatives to Hysterectomy in the Management of Leiomyomas.* Retrieved from American Congress of Obstetricians and Gynecologists: www.acog.org

Elizabeth A. Stewart, M. (2017, June 5). *Overview of treatment of uterine leiomyomas (fibroids).* Retrieved from Uptodate.com: http://uptodate.com

Geoffrey C. Cly, M. (2017, 10 27). *Expert Opinion and Current Practice Standards.* Fort Wayne, Indiana.

What I found with most patients who've had fibroids is eventually they get to a point where they come in and say, "Okay, I'm done, please take out my uterus." And for these cases, I believe they are right. It is time for a hysterectomy, this is an example, it can be a lifesaver. But, there are earlier times when they're not ready for that. Also there are women and who I see, and this is really important, I want women to know this:

If you are a woman with fibroid tumors that are growing, there will be a point in time where they grow so large that only a large painful incision is the only option, this is when a DaVinci Laparoscopy is not possible. AND when a future fertility or having babies is not possible.

Now, what do I mean by that? Well, in the case of a woman I saw recently, she had fibroids for 10 years. Her doctor, in another practice had seen her for years and was just "watching" them. Well, her largest fibroid was about six to eight centimeters and there were some other ones that were large enough to where her uterus was pushing upward and outward, almost to her belly button. By the time she came to see me, she wanted to try to get pregnant but it was too late because of how big her uterus was. The frustrating part I hear too often, is that her doctor kept telling her everything was fine and not to worry about it.

Unfortunately, in her case, she passed the point of no return. The larger fibroids completely took over her or uterus. So she didn't have any normal anatomy left and there was no way to repair the uterus. Also, when the uterus is almost all the way up to your belly button, Laparoscopic, or DaVinci is not possible because there is no room in the abdomen to visualize or navigate around the sides of the fibroids/uterus.

What I want you to know is that if you have fibroids and they are enlarging slowly they will get to a point near your uterus where you might not be able to save your uterus. If you have fibroids, I urge you to have them evaluated by a doctor who does Laparoscopic or DaVinci Myomectomies so you can develop a strategy for the future. Also, it would be recommended to get an ultrasound to find out what size they are right now so that in a year or two or three you can check you again know the rate of growth of those fibroids.

In this lady's situation, she had to have an abdominal hysterectomy and she was not able to have any more children. She did well, but she had to be in the hospital for three days. She had pain, much more pain than a DaVinci or Laparoscopic. She was not allowed to drive for two weeks and she off work for six weeks. The reality is that if she would've come in earlier, a couple of years earlier, she probably would've been able to save her uterus, go home the same day, back to work in a week, drive the next day, and have another child if she wished.

So a hysterectomy is sometimes unnecessary and sometimes a lifesaver. The research and the studies estimate about 20% of hysterectomies are unnecessary, and that's a conservative number. So what does that mean? That means that 20% of the time, or one out of five hysterectomies are unnecessary. This implies that women were not offered other procedures or treatments available to fix the problem, take care of the symptoms, and allow them to feel perfectly healthy AND save their uterus. This 20% is what I am trying to prevent. This is part of my mission.

9 Where Do We Go From Here

My hope is that you gained some insight into my world, mind, and heart but most importantly, you now realize that you have options. I hope to be able to help you along your journey to feeling healthy again and living your life to the fullest with peace, joy, and happiness.

Although this book is over 100 pages, the amount of material here is just scratching the surface. I invite you to go to HonestOBGyn.com for more information, more topics, and for any questions you might have.

When you want to become a patient and have me as your doctor and make an appointment in the office, simply go to HonestOBGyn.com, all of the contact information is available there.

When you're ready to be my client and talk to me via internet, FaceBook, live video, or through Q&A in the Members FB group then please visit my website: HonestOBGyn.com to access those options as well.

Lastly, thank you for reading or listening along to my first book. I appreciate you. I am thankful for you. I wish you happiness, health, and can't wait to meet you and to see you soon.

Truly yours,

Geoff Cly, MD, FACOG
The Honest OBGyn

ABOUT THE AUTHOR

Dr. Geoffrey Cly's college career began with visions of becoming a lawyer. It wasn't until Dr. Cly saw the documentary video "The Miracle of Life" in his general biology class that the cycle of life became a burning passion. He knew that day that his future was set. In fact, after seeing the film he changed his major and his life in medicine began.

Today Dr. Cly is a Board-Certified OB/GYN with 20 years of experience. He is one of the most experienced daVinci Robotic, Laparoscopic and Gynecological Surgeons in the Midwest with over 1000 Robotic and over 2000 laparoscopic procedures successfully performed. He has delivered over 3000 babies and seen over 100,000 patients in his 20-year career.

His passion doesn't end with his patients. As a pioneer in daVinci Minimally Invasive GYN surgery adoption that began in 2006 he became an official instructor for Intuitive, the daVinci parent company. Dr. Cly shares his knowledge and expertise by teaching most of the physicians in his region and many of the most accomplished doctors in the Midwest.

Many ask why? Why has he made it his passion to not only stay out in front of his specialty but to also teach the very doctors that could possibly be competitors? Because Dr. Cly believes women deserve to know all treatment options available and have honest, educated and up to date, physicians guiding them on their journey to health and healing. The benefits of robotic and laparoscopic surgeries allow doctors to perform complex surgeries with smaller incisions which causes less pain and allows for much quicker recoveries. This all leads to women who need less aftercare and gives them ability to get back to being productive in all aspects of their lives, mothers, caregivers, careers etc.

Dr. Cly believes all patients deserve active and competent doctors. His motto has always been "do whatever is necessary for the benefit of the patient." Each patient is a gift and his Hippocratic oath in becoming a doctor is still the most important oath of all.

Made in the USA
Columbia, SC
13 February 2021

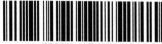